Can Humanity Survive Socialised Birth?

Dedication

PASCAL (1623–62)

'Le Coeur a ses raisons que la Raison ne connait point.'

(The heart has its reasons, of which reason knows nothing.)

21st-century interpretation:
neocortical inhibition as a key to
understanding human nature

Can Humanity Survive Socialised Birth?

Michel Odent

pinter & martin

Can Humanity Survive Socialised Birth?

First published in Great Britain by Pinter & Martin Ltd 2023

© 2023 Michel Odent

Michel Odent has asserted his moral right to be identified as the author of this work in accordance with the Copyright, Designs and Patents Act of 1988.

ISBN 978-1-78066-800-0

British Library Cataloguing-in-Publication Data
A catalogue record for this book is available from the British Library.

Set in Caslon
Printed and bound in the UK by Severn

This book has been printed on paper that is sourced and harvested from sustainable forests and is FSC accredited.

Pinter & Martin Limited
Unit 803, Omega Works
4 Roach Road
London E3 2PH

www.pinterandmartin.com

Contents

Introduction

A nonagenarian repeating himself

During conversations, people my age are often interrupted with this short sentence: 'you already told me that'. It is obvious that when our memory declines, it is easy to forget what we have recently done, said, or written. But we must also explain to younger generations that we are in a phase of our life when we feel the importance of old sayings, such as Horace's Latin *'Bis repetita placent'* – 'That which pleases is twice repeated'.

This is precisely the reason for this book. I feel the need to repeat myself. This book is an opportunity to re-evaluate the comparative importance of recently acquired insights, and to suggest links between data and ways of thinking provided by a great diversity of highly specialised disciplines.

Although each of my books has been presented with a precise focus, all of them have been about human nature, in particular about childbirth, the critical phase of human life that has been the most dramatically disrupted for millennia.

The title of this book is a question. It is premature to offer a clear conclusion. However, I find it relevant to refer to the epilogue of *Childbirth in the age of plastics*, published by Pinter & Martin in 2011. It was written to be read in 2031. Here is the last sentence:

ONLY UTOPIA CAN SAVE HUMANITY!

1

Spectacular U-turns

The 21st century can already be presented as 'the' phase of spectacular U-turns in the history of mankind. After analysing some of these concomitant U-turns, we will try to find the links between them.

Laws of natural selection
About 10 millennia ago, our ancestors started to develop their capacity to dominate Nature. This crucial worldwide phase in the history of mankind, often called the 'Neolithic revolution', included not only the domestication of plants (agriculture), and the domestication of animals (animal husbandry), but also, to a certain extent, the organisation of human life, including in particular the period surrounding birth. From that time on, human births became socialised. Concordant data about human groups that kept a palaeolithic lifestyle until the 20th century confirm that before the 'Neolithic revolution' women isolated themselves to give birth.[1,2,3]

One of the most indisputable and powerful effects of the socialisation of childbirth was to manipulate the laws of natural selection, originally by reinforcing them. The transmission from generation to generation of beliefs and rituals was an effective way to eliminate babies considered too weak to become members of the community. The most universal and surprising example of cultural interference reinforcing the selection process has been the transmission of the belief that colostrum (the 'pre-milk' secreted by the mother before her full milk supply is established) is unclean or dangerous for the baby, and that it should even be expressed and discarded.[3] At a time when we have learnt that colostrum is precious and that human babies are able to find the breast independently during the hour following birth, it is essential to interpret the quasi-universal routine of delaying the initiation of breastfeeding. Another example of such rituals is immersion in freezing water: the weakest would not survive.[4]

Furthermore, with increased socialisation, births have become increasingly difficult, and therefore more dangerous for mothers and babies. This too has enhanced the process of selection.

After millennia of enhanced selection, we have suddenly entered the era of neutralised selection. What a U-turn!

This indisputable fact has, paradoxically, attracted little attention.

It is, however, one of the main reasons to classify mankind among endangered species.

Today women who cannot give birth without medical assistance pass on their genes as easily as those who give birth by themselves. Mathematicians might already anticipate and assess the increasing difficulties of childbirth from present times.

Many recent scientific and technical advances have undoubtedly neutralised and even reversed the laws of natural selection.

For example, in the age of easy ceasarean sections, a breech presentation is hardly more dangerous, for the mother and for the baby, than a head-first presentation. Since genetic factors, transmitted by the mother and father, play an important role in the mode of presentation of the foetus,[5] this implies that in the future breech birth rates will not remain low (around 2% to 3%). They will gradually increase. The proportion of breech births in Norway was 2.5% from 1967 to 1976, 3.0% from 1977 to 1986, 3.2% from 1987 to 1996, and 3.5% from 1997 to 2004... With the data we already have, we can suggest that with appropriate computer programs it would be possible to make projections and assess the prevalence of breech presentations in a century or two. Today, being born breech means belonging to the growing fraction of the population that is very dependent on medicine (and health budgets) from the start of life.

To illustrate the almost certain effects of the neutralisation of the laws of natural selection, we can also recall that, up until now, more than 80% of human beings have belonged to the Rh-positive blood group. This fact is easily interpreted. The concept of blood incompatibility between mother and foetus helps to understand why – from a statistical perspective – an Rh-negative woman could not, until the end of the 20th century, have the same number of healthy children as an Rh-positive woman. Everything has changed since we learned how to avoid Rh incompatibility accidents by using specific agglutinins. It is therefore foreseeable – and even almost certain – that the number of Rh-negative women (and men) will now increase due to the neutralisation of the laws of natural selection. Once again, we are referring, through this example, to the growing number of humans dependent on medicine from the period around birth.

Is a 'rebirth' of the laws of natural selection impossible or utopian?

From population explosion to population implosion
The population explosion started about 10,000 years ago with the advent of agriculture and animal husbandry. During the previous 10 millennia the average temperature had risen

by at least 5 degrees Celsius, and the melting of the ice caps caused sea levels to rise by at least 100 metres. In such a climatic and geological context, the population explosion started. At the time of this 'Neolithic revolution' there were probably about 8 million human beings on Earth. Since that time this number has been multiplied by 1,000! There are currently about 8 billion humans. The word 'explosion' is justified, particularly if we consider the last 200 years. The global population was in the region of one billion around the year 1800: it had multiplied by eight within the following two centuries.

At the end of the 20th century, the population explosion was still an obsession among most policymakers and their advisers. Some of them thought the time had come to interfere urgently. The case of China is typical. China's family-planning policies began to be shaped in the 1970s, prompted by fears of overpopulation. A population planning initiative was implemented between 1980 and 2015 to curb the country's population growth by authoritatively restricting families to a single child (known as the 'one-child policy'). At the same time, in other countries, a great diversity of organisations shared the same point of view. For example, in 1974, in the UK, Family Planning Associations handed their network of over 1,000 clinics to the NHS when contraception became free for all. At the same time, in many countries, legislation about abortion was reconsidered.

Suddenly, during the years preceding the Covid-19 pandemic, a surprising powerful demographic U-turn took place. To evaluate the paramount importance of this step in the history of mankind we must keep in mind that to maintain a stable population the average number of babies per woman must be around 2.1.

Let us reconsider the case of China, as an opportunity to realise that demography is an underestimated perspective on human sexuality… and that *sexuality is outside the field of rationality.* As long as there was an anti-natalist policy (one baby per family), the population of China was paradoxically increasing. However, as soon as the politics became natalist, the average number of babies per woman started to decrease dramatically... and paradoxically. In spite of contradictions between statistics, it is probable that the number of babies per Chinese woman is not above 1.20. Interestingly, mainland China, Taiwan, Hong Kong, Singapore and South Korea are facing similar demographic issues, regardless of the apparently rational attitudes of policymakers and their advisers.

The case of South Korea is a typical example. At the start of the 1970s women had four children on average. The fertility rate in the country first dropped lower than two children per woman in 2018. Today the figure is around 0.8!

We are reaching a time when the average fertility rate across the world's most advanced economies is in the region of 1.6 children per woman. The birth implosion is well advanced all over the world, but slower in sub-Saharan Africa and countries such as Afghanistan, where the number of children per woman is still around 3.8, but continuously decreasing.

Of course, experts and the media offer simplistic rational interpretations, such as the rising cost of living, housing, childbirth, childcare and education.

Among the general public it is increasingly common to refer to 'eco-anxiety', particularly the fear of uncontrollable pollution and uncontrollable climate change. The fear of global military conflicts in the age of nuclear weapons is also increasing.

So far, statisticians have given little thought to exploring correlations between fertility rates, which have declined dramatically in a few years, and what happens during *the period surrounding birth, the critical phase of human life that has been the most profoundly modified in the 21st century.*

In the age of overspecialisation, it is difficult to keep in mind the strong physiological links between all facets of sexual reproduction: libido, sexual attraction, intercourse, pregnancy, birth process, lactation and maternal behaviour. Those who have developed an interdisciplinary perspective may already raise unprecedented questions about the recent quasi-elimination of a central phase of human reproduction. We might claim that today most women don't give birth. They are delivered by specialised experts. Women were programmed to be under the effects of specific hormonal flows. Today such hormonal flows are made redundant either by the use of substitutive pharmacology (drips of synthetic oxytocin, epidural analgesia, and so on) or by caesarean deliveries. It would be surprising if this U-turn has no statistically detectable effects on all facets of human reproductive life, and therefore on the future of our species.

At a preliminary phase, it is necessary to explore possible correlations between, on the one hand, common ways of being born in particular countries and, on the other hand, the local fertility rates. If we consider the case of China and its neighbouring countries, the very small numbers of babies per woman are associated with skyrocketing rates of caesarean section. The case of South Korea is extreme. A fecundity rate as low as 0.8 babies per woman is associated with rates of caesarean sections in the region of 50%.

There is food for thought provided by particular countries. For example, in Puerto Rico, rates of caesarean section were already as high as 31% in 1994 (the highest in the world at that time). Today the number of babies per woman is close to 1.0 (one of the lowest in the world)[6]. The case of Israel also needs to be mentioned. The number of children per woman is around 3.0 (around 6.0 among ultra-Orthodox Jews), while the rates of caesarean section are below 20%. This in turn should be compared with the case of Afghanistan, where the number of children per woman is above 3.0, with a rate of caesarean section of around 1 or 2%. In India, the most populous country in the world, both the fertility rate (2.1) and the caesarean rate (21%) are close to the global average.

If it is confirmed that there is a correlation between the way babies are born and the number of babies per woman, the next step will be to raise questions about the probability of a cause-and-effect relationship.

2

A U-turn in our understanding of human nature

Throughout the ages, a great diversity of perspectives have explored human nature and, in particular, looked at human beings in the framework of the animal kingdom. In ancient Greece, it was an objective of Aesop, via, for example, a fable such as 'The Monkey and the Dolphin': dolphins do not confuse humans with other primates. More recently, it was the objective of La Fontaine, when humanising animals in fables such as 'The Crow and the Fox'. An important step was *The classification of species* by Carl Linnaeus, written during the 18th century. The 19th century was dominated by the emergence of the theories of evolution. During the 20th century, the development of genetics has been explosive.

Since researchers sequenced the chimp genome in 2005, we have known that humans share about 99% of their DNA with chimpanzees, making them our closest living relatives. It is now thought that humans split with chimpanzees between four million and seven million years ago in Africa.[1]

This new understanding has meant that there has been a strong interest in recent years in the similarities between humans and chimpanzees. A turning point in our understanding of human nature may come when we begin to focus on the differences.

Then, we will realise that, as a general rule, our differences from the other members of the chimpanzee family are points in common with some sea mammals. An overview of these differences and common points is useful if we are to understand the particularities of human beings.

The main obvious differences are related to brain size. Brain mass in relation to the size of the body is usually quantified in terms of 'encephalisation quotient'. In humans, the encephalisation quotient (about 7.4 to 7.8) is three times higher than in the other members of the chimpanzee family (about 2.2 to 2.5).

Our selected focus: vernix caseosa

However, here we will start with the mysterious issue of vernix caseosa, because interpretations of its function have suddenly become easy and provide unexpected and irreplaceable keys to understanding human nature. Until the 21st century, in the medical and scientific literature, there was no interest in vernix caseosa. In textbooks, it was just mentioned that when human babies are born at term, their skin is covered with a kind of cream 'like cheese' (caseosa). It was also mentioned that only human babies are born with their skin covered by this cream. When I was a medical student called an 'externe' in the obstetrical department of a Paris hospital (in 1953–54) the vernix was usually wiped away. It was denied any function.

The turning point took place during the 21st century, in 2005. It was not induced by the result of a study published in a peer reviewed journal. It was due to a programme presented by David Attenborough on BBC Radio 4. The title of the programme was 'The scars of evolution'. This was when we learned that, according to Don Bowen, a marine biologist from Nova Scotia, seals are also born with their skin covered with vernix. Prior to this there had been missed opportunities to observe that sea mammals may be born with their skin covered with vernix.

In 1979 and 1981, in Western Australia, studies evaluated

the amounts of squalene in the amniotic fluid as a way to detect post-mature foetuses.[2] Squalene is an oily substance abundant among marine living creatures (the root of word squalene is *squalus*, which means shark in Latin). However, no one thought, at that time, to compare human newborn babies and the newborn babies of sea mammals. There was another missed opportunity in 2000. A team of American dermatologists wanted to develop a protective cream for premature babies. They tried to imitate vernix caseosa.[3] They were interested in 'corneocytes', which work like sponges and are protective in case of immersion in hypertonic water. However, they did not consider the case of sea mammals. In 2008 there was a study of the content of vernix caseosa focusing on branched chain fatty acids. These are special saturated fatty acids with a methyl radical (CH_3) attached to one or several carbon atoms of the molecule. Because the authors of this study had not heard about the non-published observations of seals, they could not study the vernix caseosa of sea mammals.

Finally, there was a last turning point in 2018. A team in California studied the particular case of sea lions. The authors were not aware of the observations by Don Bowen about seals. Foetuses of sea lions also have their skin covered with human-like vernix.[4] At the end of pregnancy, particles of vernix become detached from the skin and enrich the amniotic fluid. This is how the foetuses of sea lions and humans swallow molecules of branched chain fatty acids that probably play an important role in the way the gut flora is established. It will be important to study in depth the similarities between humans and sea mammals in terms of development of the gut flora. Meanwhile, let us first keep in mind that, with its corneocytes, vernix caseosa is protective in the case of immersion in (hypertonic) sea water.

Beyond our selected focus

There are many other reasons to present humans as a kind of 'marine chimpanzee'. One of them is the need for iodine. Most human beings, if they don't have easy access to the seafood chain, cannot consume a sufficient amount of iodine. It is the most common nutritional deficiency in the world, at such a point that many governments have established regulations so that table salt is enriched with iodine. It is a common issue in pregnant and lactating women, who need about 1.5 times the normal amount of iodine.

We know why this is serious. *Homo* is characterised by a huge brain. The development and functions of the brain are highly dependent on thyroid hormones. Iodine is necessary for their synthesis. The American Thyroid Association (ATA) claims that pregnant women should take a daily iodine supplement of 150μg. According to a British study, when pregnant women take such a supplement, the average IQ of their children is multiplied by 1.22.[5] So, when we consider the most common nutritional deficiency among modern humans, we are tempted to associate the terms marine and chimpanzee when referring to our species.

The brain is a fatty organ. This implies that it has specific needs in term of lipids. It has, in particular, a specific need for DHA (docosahexaenoic acid). DHA is a molecule of omega-3 fatty acid that is as long and as desaturated as possible (22 carbons and six double bonds). The point is that the human enzymatic system is not very effective in synthesizing DHA, which is preformed and abundant only in the seafood chain.[6–8] If human beings don't have access to seafood their enzymatic system (desaturase and elongase) must transform the parent molecule of the omega-3 family (only 18 carbons and three double bonds), which is provided by the land food chain. The point is that this enzymatic system is not very effective in humans. This is one of the most mysterious aspects of human nature: the highly developed brain needs the fatty acid DHA, but the human enzymatic system is not very effective at synthetising this molecule, which is preformed in the seafood chain. Enzymes need the help of catalysts, mostly minerals provided by the land food chain. The point is that this metabolic pathway is fragile. It can be weakened by emotional states associated with the release of corticosteroids, such as being sad or depressed, and by potential inhibitory factors such as the consumption of pure sugar, alcohol, trans fatty acids, and man-made food in general. Ideally, we probably need to consume fatty acids abundant in the seafood chain.

A reference to our enzymatic system is providing another reason to develop the concept of 'marine'. There are very aquatic mammals that do not have access to a marine environment, for example water voles, otters, rhinoceroses, elephants and hippopotami. We don't have many common points with them. When we claim that we are special compared with other mammals, we find reasons to emphasise our common points with sea mammals rather than aquatic mammals in general, since our main particularity is expressed in terms of encephalisation quotient.

There are many other differences between human beings and chimpanzees. It is worth mentioning them, although none of them has the power to undermine the dominant theoretical framework.

- Nakedness
- The direction in which the hairs lie on different parts of the body
- A subcutaneous layer of fat
- Bipedalism – a heavy head is incompatible with all types of quadrupedalism. On the other hand, bipedal humans can even add weights on their head while walking. Normal humans may be considered 'obligate' full-time bipeds because the alternatives are very uncomfortable

and usually only resorted to when walking is impossible.

• Attitude to the placenta – it seems that in our species 'placentophagy', the consumption of the placenta by the mother immediately after birth, as is observed in numerous terrestrial mammals, has never been instinctive.[9,10] If it had been at any time in the history of humanity, we would find traces of this behaviour in myths, legends, and reports from preliterate and preagricultural societies. I know of women who have reached a very instinctive state of consciousness in the perinatal period, behaving as if 'on another planet', and overcoming a great part of their cultural conditioning. Yet none of them ever expressed a tendency to bring the placenta toward her mouth.[13] Modern women who have occasionally eaten pieces of placenta have been inspired by theories such as the idea that it might prevent postnatal depression. Scientific interest in the placenta has recently inspired such theories, leading to a form of human placentophagy based on rational considerations. For example, the discovery by Kristal of a placental substance that makes endorphins more effective ('Placental Opioid-Enhancing Factor') could be seen as a justification for placentophagy in our species.[11] However, we should avoid the conclusion that eating placenta is an innate human behaviour. Exploring placentophagy is important since, as a general rule, land mammals eat the placenta. If eating the placenta has never been instinctive among our ancestors, this would be another common point with sea mammals, including carnivorous cetaceans and seals. Interestingly, camels are the exceptions among land mammals: they do not eat the placenta. Camels have another particularity among land mammals: like *Homo* and sea mammals they have kidneys with medullary pyramids. Since camels consume highly salty plants and drink the water of salty ponds, and since sea mammals also have easy access to hypertonic salty substances, placentophagy might be correlated with an urgent need for specific nutrients, particularly minerals, in the postpartum period. It is as if placentophagy and non-pyramidal renal medullas were features shared by mammals that do not have access to hypertonic salty substances after parturition. Can camels from the desert help us to accept our coastal origins?

- The sense of smell of human beings is mysteriously weak. It is the same among whales. When they separated from hoofed mammals about 60 million years ago and migrated to water, their sense of smell nearly disappeared.

- Body temperature control through the loss of sweat is not a costly mechanism if we think of the human being as a primate adapted to environments where water and minerals are available without restriction. The density of sweat glands among humans is 10 times higher than among chimpanzees. Interestingly, fur seals sweat through abundant eccrine glands when they are overheated on land.

- A low larynx, which gives us the ability to breathe through our nose or our mouth, is an anatomical particularity shared with sea lions and dugongs.

- A prominent nose is a feature shared with proboscis monkeys, the most marine of the primates, which live in coastal wetlands in Borneo. They are bipedal. They are excellent distance swimmers. They are able to swim 20 metres under water. Their toes are webbed.

- The human vagina, like that of sea mammals, is long and oblique.

- The human apolipoprotein E gene has more similarities with that of sea mammals than that of land mammals (including common chimpanzees and bonobos).[12] Apolipoprotein E is the principal cholesterol carrier in the brain.

- Growth of bone in the ear canal is particular to modern humans who are frequent swimmers, and seals, as mammals adapted to both underwater life and life on dry land. 'External auditory exostoses' are dense bony growths protruding into the ear canal at two or three constant sites. It is notable that they were first described in 1911 by Marcellin Boule in his classic monograph on the Neanderthal skeleton from the Bouffia Bonneval in La Chapelle-aux-Saints, France.[13] Since that time, it has been confirmed that the Neanderthals exhibited an exceptionally high level of auditory exostosis: in the region of 50%.[14] We must keep in mind that Neanderthals had enormous brains and, probably, a special relationship with water, since they could be skilled long-distance navigators. Today the colloquial term for these exostoses is 'surfer's ear' because, among modern humans, it is usually associated with frequent swimming and water immersion of the auditory canal. Many water sports have developed recently. This is a reason why 'surfer's ear' is becoming so topical in the specialised medical literature, and that some common beliefs are suddenly being reconsidered. For example, a study assessed surfers living and surfing in Queensland, Australia.[15] It appeared that in young to quadragenarian-aged warm-water surfers, the prevalence and severity of auditory exostosis were much higher than anticipated: it had previously only been shown to occur in cold-water surfers. This is in agreement with a report by Nicole Smith-Guzmán, who found seven cases of surfer's ear in males and one in a female skull in an ancient burial ground in a pre-Columbian village near the Gulf of Panama, at an equatorial latitude.[16] In such a renewed scientific context, Peter Rhys-Evans suggested that aural exostoses were evolved during a certain phase of the history of mankind for protection of the delicate tympanic membrane during swimming and diving by narrowing the ear canal in a similar fashion to other semiaquatic species.[17]

- One of the most common abnormalities (or particularities) in humans is webbing between the second and the third toe. When a congenital abnormality is an addition, it usually means that the feature was there for a reason during the evolutionary process.
- A narrowing of the thoracic aorta ('coarctation of the aorta') is common among humans and seals.
- Menopause, and prolonged life after reproduction, is a feature shared by humans, killer whales and short-finned pilot whales.

By focusing on the main differences between *Homo* and the other members of the chimpanzee family, we have radically reconsidered the comparative importance of some indisputable and highly significant characteristics of human beings. For example, we found great significance in the creamy substance that covers the skin of the newborn of some sea mammals and humans since, undoubtedly, it is protective in case of immersion in hypertonic water such as sea water. We also attached special importance to the most common human nutritional deficiency in the world: lack of iodine, which is a serious issue in the case of pregnant women and lactating mothers. We also considered that the defining feature of *Homo* is a supersized brain. Our objective is not to inspire new theories. Theories can have negative effects – they 'freeze' our ways of thinking and prevent us from thinking more broadly and continuing to pose important questions. During the 21st century, several emerging and fast-developing scientific disciplines have arisen precisely to initiate new ways of thinking, rather than discussing the content of established theories.

Until now, in our studies of human nature, and particularly of the differences between *Homo* and chimpanzees, we have purposely remained in the framework of anatomy and physiology. We shall not go beyond this framework now, because it would lead us to raise countless further questions about the complex issues of human sociability and human adaptability. How do we explain that only members of our species can adapt to all latitudes, from the equator to the polar areas? How do we explain that members of our species can adapt to both sea level and high altitudes? How can we adapt to a great diversity of food? There is no end to the questions we could explore.

3

'If you consume the fruit of the tree of knowledge… in sorrow you'll give birth'

This message, written thousands of years ago, has been transmitted from generation to generation… until the time when an interpretation could be offered. We have reached that time.

It is highly significant that the Bible – as an enormous library about the lifestyle of our ancestors after they learnt to dominate Nature – starts with two related priority topics: the handicap of knowing too much, and the difficulties of human births. I'll translate and explain in modern scientific language what our contemporaries need to assimilate. This is the core – the 'main dish' – of my oral and written messages as a nonagenarian.

Up until now, the common question 'Why are human births difficult?' has been answered with 'It is for mechanical reasons'. Such replies have often been justified by pictures comparing the size and shape of the maternal pelvis with the size and shape of the foetal head. There has been no need for long paragraphs of explanation, since it is impossible to modify the bony pelvis of a pregnant woman. This is why, in textbooks, chapters about birth physiology in humans are short.

It will be another matter when it becomes commonplace

to wonder: 'Why are human births occasionally easy?' Even in the 21st century, we have all heard about women who, surprisingly, gave birth very easily and quickly. Such anecdotes suggest that, until now, there has been a tendency to overestimate the importance of mechanical factors.

When the tool becomes the master

Remember that a gigantic brain, and in particular a highly developed 'new brain' (the neocortex), is what makes members of our species different from all other mammals. In a renewed scientific context, we are in a position to understand that the neocortex does not always play the role of a tool at the service of physiological functions. It can be the opposite. When a human behaviour or a human physiological function has mysterious characteristics, we must keep in mind that the activity of the powerful new brain can have inhibitory effects: 'the tool can become the master'. We have a lot to learn from the multiple examples of human physiological functions that are easily obscured by neocortical activity.

The sense of smell, apparently weak in adult humans, is a typical example. An ingenious sophisticated experiment has eloquently demonstrated that the human sense of smell is improved following alcohol consumption. It is well known that alcohol reduces inhibition.[1] It is highly significant that olfaction appears as an important physiological function in newborn babies until a certain degree of neocortical development. I highlighted as early as the 1970s that, immediately after birth, it is mostly through the sense of smell that the baby is guided towards the nipple.[2,3] Since that time, there has been an intense curiosity, in scientific circles, about the functions of the sense of smell in early infancy.[4-12] One of the reasons for this curiosity is that the sense of smell becomes gradually weaker after the first few weeks following birth. The concept of neocortical inhibition offers the most valuable interpretation.

It is also worth recalling that in all human societies, even those where genital sexuality is comparatively free, couples isolate themselves to make love. Such a universally accepted need for privacy in specific situations indicates a deep-rooted understanding of an essential aspect of human nature.

Until now, the concept of neocortical inhibition has not been commonly mentioned by medical practitioners, apart from psychiatrists: in the particular case of pathological conditions associated with culturally unacceptable behaviours, there is evidence for impaired inhibition. However, although not often mentioned, the concept is understood in an empiric way by some clinicians. For example, a urologist specialised in prostatic diseases would never ask a man to urinate in front of him to evaluate the power of his urine jet.

It is artificial to separate the issue of neocortical inhibition from the issue of 'primitive reflexes'. These reflex actions are exhibited by normal infants, but disappear after some weeks or months and are not exhibited by normal adults. The 'rooting reflex', thanks to which a newborn baby can find the breast during the hour following birth, is usually mentioned in this framework. From a theoretical perspective, the important point is that older children and adults with pathological conditions such as cerebral palsy may retain these reflexes. Furthermore, such reflexes may reappear in neurological conditions such as dementia, strokes, and after traumatic lesions. It is also significant that primitive reflexes can reappear among normal elderly people: this is an obvious sign of the physiological ageing of the neocortex and its declining inhibitory power.[13]

When the concept of neocortical inhibition is assimilated, those who wonder why human births are occasionally easy will be ready to understand that reduced neocortical control is nature's solution.

The solution found by nature

Even during the 21st century, there are still people who know that when a woman is giving birth easily, there comes a time when she appears to cut herself off from our world. She forgets what she has been taught, what she read in books, and what her plans were. She may behave in a way that would usually be considered unbecoming to 'civilised' women, for example screaming or swearing. She may complain about odours nobody else can perceive. She may find herself in the most unexpected and bizarre primitive postures, often quadrupedal. Reduced neocortical activity can explain the well-known fact that many women forget details of what happened when they were in labour. Hundreds of women were interviewed about 10 days after giving birth. Those who had given birth by caesarean had a comparatively good recollection of many details.[14]

In a renewed scientific context, this is how we can summarise the basic needs of a labouring woman: she needs to feel protected against all possible neocortical stimulations. The keyword here is 'protected'. Since language is a powerful neocortical stimulant, it is easy to reach the conclusion that silence is a basic need. One of the effects of the socialisation of childbirth, as an aspect of the domination of Nature that started about 10,000 years ago, has been to increase the risks of being exposed to language during labour. Of course, there are differences between several kinds of language in terms of neocortical stimulation. There are differences between a language absorbed during foetal life and infancy versus a language learned as a university student. We may contrast baby language and intellectualised language. Asking a question is always a powerful way to stimulate neocortical activity. *I have suggested that 'in the land of Utopia' the capacity to remain silent would be a prime criterion for being accepted as a midwifery student.*

The effects of light on the birth process have not been

taken seriously until recently, when it became apparent that melatonin, the 'darkness hormone', is an essential birth hormone. This is why it is worth focusing on this factor. Studies of the interactions between melatonin and other brain mediators offer a promising avenue for research. The effects of melatonin as an inhibitor of neocortical activity are already well understood.[15,16] We feel obliged to deviate from the concept of neocortical inhibition and refer to recent advances in our knowledge of the peripheral effects of melatonin. It is now established that there are melatonin receptors in the human uterus, and that melatonin works together with oxytocin to enhance the contractility of uterine muscle.[17-21]

The point is that melatonin appears today to be an important hormonal agent in human birth. This is confirmed by the significant amount of melatonin in the blood of neonates, except those born by pre-labour caesarean.[22] The importance of these findings is clearly seen when the protective anti-oxidative properties of melatonin are taken into account. In the age of artificial lights, reasons to improve our understanding of melatonin release and the properties of melatonin become obvious. We must realise that we are at a turning point in the history of light. Until recently the emission of light was based on the phenomenon of incandescence: sun, fire, classical electrical bulbs, and so on. Today, light-emitting diodes (LEDs) are semiconductor sources emitting light comparatively rich in the blue spectrum. It is already well established that this part of the spectrum is the most melatonin suppressive. The need to illuminate a birthing place is an effect of the socialisation of the event.

As a general rule, we just need to keep in mind that all attention-enhancing situations stimulate neocortical activity and therefore inhibit the birth process. Feeling observed is a typical example of this kind of situation: in other words, privacy appears to be a basic need. The perception of possible danger is another typical situation: in other words, feeling secure also appears to be a basic need.

After such considerations about what can make a human birth possible and even occasionally easy, we are in a position to describe and interpret the phase of preparation for what is known as 'the foetus ejection reflex'. A labouring woman may suddenly talk nonsense, as if she were on another planet. After thousands of years of socialisation of childbirth and cultural conditioning, it is rare that an authentic foetus ejection reflex can follow. However, it is possible.

The foetus ejection reflex

I am often asked to clarify the difference between the foetus ejection reflex and the Ferguson's reflex. In around 1940, when working with anaesthetised rabbits, Ferguson studied uterine contractions induced by vaginal dilation.[23] It was demonstrated afterwards that in parturient sheep the 'Ferguson reflex' is associated with increased blood concentrations of oxytocin and utero-ovarian venous prostaglandin-F levels.[24] It was also demonstrated that these responses are blocked by epidural anesthesia.[25] The results of such studies, focusing on vaginal dilation, immediately attracted the attention of those in medical circles.

Niles Newton, on the other hand, looked at the effects of environmental factors on the birth of mice. By focusing on the importance of cortical inhibition, even among non-human mammals, she was studying parturition as a chapter of brain physiology.[26] She used the term 'foetus ejection reflex'. It is significant that, compared with the work of Ferguson, the studies by Niles Newton have not attracted the same attention within obstetrical circles.

In the 1980s, I suggested that an authentic foetus ejection reflex is also possible in humans, but is usually repressed by neocortical activity. With the support of Niles

Newton, I wrote that saving this term from oblivion would be key to facilitating a radically new understanding of the particularities of human parturition.[27,28] I had observed that, in exceptionally rare situations, women do experience this reflex after a short series of irresistible and powerful contractions that precede the baby's birth. In such situations, voluntary movement has no place. When a typical reflex occurs, there is an obvious elimination of neocortical control: women seem to be 'on another planet', talking nonsense, behaving in a way usually considered unacceptable for civilised women, and finding themselves in the most unexpected, bizarre, often mammalian bending forward or quadrupedal postures. The reflex does not always start at the same phase of descent of the foetal presenting part. A real foetus ejection reflex can occur long before the descent of the presenting part, or long after. It can start before complete dilation or after complete dilation. At the very moment of the birth, mothers are typically in an ecstatic state: they may need some time to realise that the baby is born and dare to take him or her in their arms.

It is easy to explain why the concept of foetus ejection reflex is not well understood after thousands of years of socialisation of childbirth. It is precisely when delivery seems to be imminent that the birth attendant tends to become even more intrusive. The foetus ejection reflex can be preceded by sudden, explosive expression of a fear with a frequent reference to death.[29] Any attempt to reassure with words can interrupt progress towards the foetus ejection reflex.[30] In the particular context of a preliterate and pre-agricultural society in New Guinea, Wulf Schiefenhovel could discreetly film women giving birth in the bush, without any assistance, through authentic foetus ejection reflexes similar to those some modern women occasionally experience in ideal situations.[31] In general, any interference tends to bring the labouring woman 'back down to Earth' and tends to transform the foetus ejection reflex into a second stage of labour which involves voluntary movements.

Today, there is no simple recipe to overcome thousands of years of cultural conditioning. However, I can describe an environment, at the limit of utopia in the case of civilised modern women, that is compatible with an authentic foetus ejection reflex. The reflex is more likely to occur in a small dark room at a comfortable ambient temperature, with no one around.

The popularisation of the concept of the foetus ejection reflex, as a consequence of a renewed understanding of birth physiology, would be a critical step towards a certain degree of desocialisation of childbirth. Can we present authentic midwifery as the art of *protecting* an environment compatible with a foetus ejection reflex?

Interaction between two pure mammals

When we use the phrase 'pure mammal' about our species, we have in mind phases of human life that are not powerfully controlled by neocortical activity. The most typical example is the interaction between a mother and her newborn immediately after a foetus ejection reflex. As the reflex could be expressed, this implies that the maternal neocortex is at rest. The baby is then in an early phase of neocortical development, and their 'archaic reflexes' can be highlighted. When these maternal and neonatal reflexes are not inhibited, humans have more similarities with other mammals. This interaction between two 'pure mammals' is difficult to understand after millennia of socialised childbirth. Today the need for voluntary muscular efforts is usual during an 'expulsive period' (the second phase of labour).

It is worth observing and emphasising that since the domination of Nature that defined the 'Neolithic revolution', the crucial phase of 'interaction between two pure mammals' has been radically suppressed under the effect of cultural conditioning constantly reinforced by the transmission from generation to generation of beliefs and rituals. When I was a medical student in the mid-20th century, newborns were not 'allowed' to find the breast until they were two or three days old. The cultural environment forbade the interaction between 'two pure mammals'. The day we accept that the role of the authentic midwife is to protect an environment compatible with the foetus ejection reflex, is the day when we will be able to challenge thousands of years of tradition. Then we will realise that, from the very first minutes after birth, not only does the newborn need its mother, but also that the mother needs the newborn. The interaction takes place in particular through skin-to-skin contact, the perception of odours, the meeting of gazes and vocal exchanges. This interaction facilitates the release of a huge surge of maternal oxytocin, allowing delivery of the placenta without dangerous blood loss. A big step will be taken when it is understood that childbirth, and in particular the foetus ejection reflex, is part of a physiological preparation for breastfeeding.

After thousands of years of tradition

By studying childbirth in the light of modern physiology, we challenge thousands of years of cultural conditioning. We present the process of childbirth as an involuntary process under the control of primitive brain structures that we share with other mammals. As a rule, we cannot help an involuntary process, but we can identify inhibiting factors. From a practical point of view, in terms of basic needs, let us consider 'protection'. Since our starting point is the concept of neocortical inhibition, protection from language was privileged. If our starting point had been the concept of adrenaline-oxytocin antagonism in mammals in general, we would have first mentioned protection from low ambient temperatures and from fear-inducing situations. Just keep in mind that in general, when mammals release emergency hormones of the adrenaline family, they cannot release oxytocin, the main hormone of childbirth. As a rule, in emergency situations, mammals postpone physiological processes related to reproduction, while they need energy to fight or flee.

This reference to adrenaline-oxytocin antagonism is an opportunity to recall that in the middle of the 20th century, when I was a medical student in the obstetrics department of a Paris hospital, the midwives spent their lives knitting. At the April 2004 British Psychological Society conference, Emily Holmes presented her studies on the effects of repetitive tasks, such as knitting, in stressful situations.[32] The author could conclude from her studies that repetitive tasks are an effective way to affect emotional states. Emily Holmes pointed out that her research was consistent with the behaviours of the famous knitters of the French Revolution, such as Madame Defarges, who were knitting while watching the condemned being guillotined. These knitters, apparently, were not at risk of post-traumatic stress disorder. Emily Holmes also referred to the use of 'worry beads' in many cultures, such as Greece, as a way of coping with stressful situations.

We could translate these observations into physiological language and realise that when midwives spend long hours knitting, their own adrenaline levels are kept as low as possible. Since high levels of adrenaline are extremely contagious, the progress of labour depends largely on the physiological balance of those who, for socio-cultural reasons, might feel compelled to be present.[33,34] What is the future of knitting in midwifery schools?

Introducing 'protection' as a keyword is a simple and concise way to challenge tradition. Since the beginning of the socialisation of childbirth as a component of the domination of Nature, one of the bases of our conditioning has been that a woman does not have the power to give birth by herself. She needs various cultural interferences. The dominant paradigm has gone through many phases, from the advent of the midwife and perinatal beliefs and rituals to the masculinisation and medicalisation of the environment. Current keywords always emphasise the active role of someone other than the mother and baby, the two obligatory actors in the event. They are variants of the concepts of helping and controlling. The terms 'coaching', used by groups promoting 'natural childbirth', and 'labour management', used in medical circles, imply the intervention of an expert, while the term 'support' suggests that to give birth a woman needs energy brought by somebody else.

When the term 'protection' prevails over the current keywords, we will have reached a vital turning point in our understanding of human birth.

4

In the age of the sorcerer's apprentices

Over the past decades humanity has accumulated and shared an enormous amount of scientific knowledge at an unprecedented rate. Today, there is an urgent need to learn how to use what has been acquired.

How can we overcome the effects of the extreme dispersion of available knowledge in the age of hyperspecialisation? It is relatively easy to acquire fragmented knowledge. What is difficult is to change one's way of thinking in a renewed scientific context; to make syntheses; to formulate questions adapted to unprecedented situations; to detect 'a needle in a haystack'.

We have already given examples of the need to reformulate old questions in order to learn to use knowledge from emerging scientific disciplines. We have pointed out, for example, that instead of constantly asking why human births are difficult, it becomes more fruitful in the era of modern neurophysiology to ask why births are occasionally quick and easy.

Because the transition from knowledge to awareness should be one of the great concerns of our time, we are led to mention questions that one only thinks of formulating if the perspective is interdisciplinary. Here are two examples.

1. When did the 'epidemic' of labour induction begin?

It is increasingly common in modern obstetrics to shorten the duration of foetal life through interventions such as induction of labour and caesarean section before labour begins. This is a reason to gather data that has so far been poorly collated, firstly because it is scattered, and secondly because *its importance cannot be evaluated as long as the human capacity to think long term is not widely developed.* Only a synthesis of useful acquired knowledge can make us aware of the importance of a short 'physiological preparation phase for labour'.[1]

It is precisely at a time when we are acquiring valuable information about this phase that experts provide guidelines that are probably responsible, to a certain extent, for the current epidemic of labour induction.

Joint Spanish/Dutch brain imaging studies have revealed that in late pregnancy specific areas of grey matter involved in socialisation decrease in volume. It is as if the need for privacy precedes the onset of labour to some extent.[2] Another aspect of this physiological preparation is an increase in blood melatonin concentrations. Let us keep in mind the synergies between melatonin and oxytocin, and between melatonin and mediators that inhibit neocortical activity.[3,4]

These scattered data on maternal physiology become important when combined with data provided by experts in placental physiology. In late pregnancy, the placenta produces a peak of 'ALLO' (for allopregnanolone), a substance that acts as a moderator of neocortical activity.[5]

In such a context, we are led to rescue from oblivion some epidemiological data that have gone unnoticed despite their great scientific value and possible practical implications. A Swedish study found that the longer a boy has been in the womb, the lower his risk of prostate cancer in old age. The investigation involved a huge cohort of men born in Stockholm between 1889 and 1941 and 834 cases of prostate cancer were identified in this group between 1958 and 1994.[6] The reasons why such a study went unnoticed are easily understood in the current phase of the history of information technology. For one thing, it was published in a serious scientific journal which was too specialised to be read by practitioners. Moreover, even if the article had reached some practitioners, it is likely that most would not have gone beyond the title: prostate cancer experts have little interest in the length of foetal life, and gynaecologists and midwives are not conditioned to think long-term and take an interest in prostate cancers.

To complete this illustration of the irreplaceable power of interdisciplinary perspectives, I will mention again what I learned from reading an article on human-like vernix caseosa...in sea lions.[7] I became aware that the vernix particles that are shed from the skin of the foetus and suspended in the amniotic fluid are swallowed and participate in the development of the intestinal flora. The importance of the intestinal flora in the way health is organised is becoming increasingly well understood. The phase of preparation for labour is also a phase of preparation for extra-uterine life for the baby. We understand why sorcerer's apprentices ignore it.

These considerations about artificially shortened pregnancies lead us to recall that the most common alleged reason for labour induction is the fear of foetal distress related to prolonged pregnancy: the main guide is the calendar providing information about gestational age. It would be more rational to evaluate placental function. If there was frequent demand, many laboratories would be in a position to quickly measure the concentrations of placental hormones in the urine of the mother. Through this strategy, I learnt that some babies seem to be perfectly mature before 40 weeks of gestation, while others need a much longer time. Employing this testing strategy would dramatically reduce the number of labour inductions.

2. When did agriculture start?

While human beings endowed with a powerful brain appeared hundreds of thousands of years ago, any student of human nature is entitled to wonder why, during a period reduced to a few millennia which began about 10,000 years ago, our ancestors suddenly domesticated plants and animals and developed agriculture. The quasi-synchronicity of the advent of agriculture (and other aspects of the domination of Nature) on the five continents, among populations who could not communicate, is *a priori* mysterious. Of course, there were variations in the nature of the plants grown depending on the geological and climatic context.

In the Near East, for example, the cultivation of wheat, barley and rye began very early and then spread to southwest Asia and Europe. In most of the Asian continent, rice and millet cultivation began at about the same time, as did taro cultivation in New Guinea. As far as the New World is concerned, it is accepted that it was in Mesoamerica that the cultivation of plants such as corn, beans and squash began.

This synchronicity in the advent of agriculture is mysterious, except to those who understand that any study of a phase of *Homo*'s evolution requires reference to the evolution of 'Planet Ocean' during the same period. An interdisciplinary perspective requires us to recall that the last ice age reached its peak about 20,000 years ago. The average temperature was then about 6°C. Over the next 10,000 years, the average temperature rose by at least 5°C, and the melting of the ice caps led to a rise in sea levels of at least 100 metres. In some regions, the effects of rising sea levels have been dramatic. For example, in the southern Mediterranean part of the Iberian Peninsula, the shoreline is estimated to have moved 140 metres every 50 years, which is noticeable in a human lifetime. This means that the surface of the continental zones has decreased considerably. This explains why human populations all over the world have adapted to the rapid evolution of the planet by radically transforming their lifestyles. These lifestyle changes were based on agriculture, but also on animal husbandry and other aspects of the domination of Nature, such as, in the human species, the organisation of physiological processes related to reproduction. *The domination of Nature preceded the development of the capacity for long-term thinking. This explains the advent of the sorcerer's apprentice.*

Our interpretations of the 'Neolithic revolution' are not based on the acquisition of scientific data that is still confidential. We have simply emphasised the importance of interdisciplinary perspectives in moving from established knowledge to awareness.

Can sorcerer's apprentices be neutralised?
A synthesis of the knowledge we have at our disposal today could make it possible, to a certain extent, to prevent or neutralise worrying behaviours.

It is urgent to disclose the multiple emerging scientific data likely to protect *Homo* and Planet Ocean against sorcerer's apprentices trapped in short-term thinking. *Homo* – the primate endowed with a powerful neocortical supercomputer – has an immense capacity to leap from one order of magnitude to another. Until recently, the development of this capacity was not considered an essential component in educational programmes.

Should the development of the capacity to jump from one scale to another become an important topic for all interdisciplinary students in human nature?

The answer is undoubtedly 'yes', even if we do not take into account the power of 21st-century medicine.

For example, we learn from some scientists that the diameter of an atom of helium is about 0.06 nanometres. A nanometre is one billionth of a metre (0.00000000m). At the same time, we can learn that the distance from the

Earth to the edge of the visible universe is about 45.7 billion light-years. A light year is equivalent to about 9.46 trillion kilometres.

Where evaluation of time is concerned, we need milliseconds as a unit when studying liquid-crystal displays (LCDs) that have a wide range of applications. A millisecond is a thousandth of a second. In contrast, we must be able to think in terms of hundreds of thousand years when considering the protection of an ecosystem against nuclear waste, while we need to think in terms of billions of years when referring to the history of life on Earth.

The turning point in the history of the relationship between *Homo* and space and time is symbolised by the work of Galileo, during the 17th century. The term 'microscope' was coined in 1625, when Galileo presented a new instrument to the Accademia dei Lincei that made visible objects that were imperceptible to the naked eye. At the same time Galileo, as the 'Father of observational astronomy', pointed a telescope skyward. He was able to discern mountains and craters on the moon, as well as a ribbon of diffuse light arching across the sky – the Milky Way. He also discovered the rings of Saturn, sunspots and four of Jupiter's moons.

Before this turning point, the human capacity to scale change had already appeared as an essential aspect of human nature. Objects resembling lenses date back 4,000 years and there are Greek accounts from the 5th century BC of the optical properties of water-filled spheres.

A 32,500-year-old carved ivory mammoth tusk could contain the oldest known star chart (resembling the constellation Orion).[9] Where the relationship with time is concerned, it is worth noticing that there were Sumerian, Egyptian, Assyrian and Elamite calendars.

Interdisciplinary perspectives imply the capacity to adapt to a great diversity of orders of magnitude. Our study of the relationship between *Homo* and water led us to introduce issues such as the colonisation of the Pacific Rim by '*Homo Navigator*'. My dormant interest in '*Homo* and water' was awakened in the age of tap water by objects... the size of a garden paddling pool.

The answer to our question about the development of the capacity to think long-term is also an unequivocal 'yes' if we consider the case of medicine, and particularly reproductive medicine involving humans with a life expectancy of about 80 years. Why are we not more curious about the possible long-term consequences of being born under the effects of drips of synthetic oxytocin, or modern techniques of epidural anaesthesia, or by prelabour caesarean section, or after receiving antibiotics? Questions of this type are why I set up the Primal Health Research Database, which I began to populate in 1986.[8]

5

The future of the shamanic midwife

In the age of standardisation

One of the most recent, spectacular and risky feats of the 'sorcerer's apprentices' is the quasi-standardisation of an obstetrical strategy based on 'substitutive pharmacology'. This means in particular that the release of natural oxytocin – a hormone well known for its mechanical effects on the uterine muscle – is now easily replaced by intravenous infusions of synthetic oxytocin. This also means that natural opiates (the 'endorphins') are replaced by synthetic opiates injected preferably into the epidural space. Since in our cultural circles it is not usual to move away from short-term concerns, discussions are focused on details, without questioning the dominant strategies. It is easy to ignore information that might challenge standard ways of thinking limited to the short term.[1]

This is worth thinking about, because a newborn baby is a human being with a life expectancy of about 80 years, and we are now in a position to assert – if we dare to take into consideration disturbing data – that during a critical phase of development, the brain of a human foetus is under the effect of high concentrations of synthetic oxytocin. On the one hand, the concentrations of oxytocin in the maternal blood must be very high to compensate for the fact that its release is not pulsatile. On the other hand, placental enzymes are not in practice powerful enough to neutralise oxytocin.[2] It is also well known that the protective 'blood-brain' barrier is not functional before birth.

To point out that today most babies born vaginally – as well as most of those born by caesarean section after a vaginal birth attempt – are exposed to high concentrations of oxytocin is to realise the importance of the subject with regards to the future of the human species. Similar comments could be made about modern epidurals with synthetic opiate injections, for which only medium-term studies are available regarding the quality and duration of breastfeeding.

It appears that modern epidurals with opiates are more disruptive to breastfeeding than traditional epidurals with only local anesthetics.[3]

While there is an urgent need for long-term thinking, useful studies are already theoretically possible. I have suggested the use of physiological clocks, and in particular epigenetic clocks.[4] The principle of these clocks is based on the fact that each human being has two ages that can be compared. The chronological age, which is very precise, takes into account only the date of birth. The physiological age takes into account the fact that certain bodily functions evolve throughout the human life. This is one aspect of the ageing process. By studying how certain genes are educated, under certain circumstances, not to express themselves, we can to some extent assess physiological age. Because synthetic oxytocin infusions have been widely used for half a century and epidurals with opiates since the end of the 20th century, the priority is to be aware of what is at stake. Until a new generation of studies is available, great caution should be the basis of any strategy. In some situations, an attitude dominated by the 'precautionary principle' may suggest, for example, that it is better for the foetus and the mother to opt for an elective caesarean section during labour, rather than to initiate a lengthy phase of pharmacological assistance.

An analysis of one of the characteristics of modern

obstetrics leads to the point that the typical modern midwife can be presented as a technician educated to follow protocols.

The shamanic attitude

Having implied that in the age of substitutive pharmacology 'love hormones' have become redundant in the period around birth, and while the concept of neocortical inhibition becomes a key to understanding certain physiological functions in the human species, it is inevitable to mention what we call, for simplicity, the shamanic attitude. The shamanic attitude is, to some extent, the opposite of the currently dominant attitude. It concerns physiological functions that are more or less inhibited by neocortical activity. The prototype of such functions is childbirth. The objective, which is easy to explain in the 21st century, is not to replace hormonal mediators. It is to facilitate their release.

This leads me to talk about how, in 1964, I suddenly understood what characterises childbirth in the human species, and how I developed an interest in shamanic attitudes. I had the opportunity to realise that incantations and the transmission of transcendent emotional states by contagion were only components of the shamanic attitude and that the relative importance of psychedelic substances was often underestimated.

At a time when bureaucratic imperatives were simplified, a friend of mine, a doctor working for a pharmaceutical company, gave me some samples of a recently synthesised substance called Gamma-Hydroxybutyric Acid (GHB). In the context of the 1960s he was already able to explain that it was an analogue of GABA (Gamma-Aminobutyric Acid), which could not be dangerous because it was an integral part of the mammalian central nervous system.[5] This newly marketed substance was presented as a sedative drug with a promising future in anaesthesiology. My friend added that, according to several preliminary reports, it also shared the properties of oxytocin.

This is how I experienced a few deliveries with infusions of what was called in France gamma-OH. With such infusions, the women completely lost their minds, screaming in the corridors, tearing out the intravenous needle, frightening the midwife...but the baby was born in a very short time. Of course, such scenes were unacceptable in a hospital environment, and we had to be careful about possible negative side effects that hindsight could bring to light. The main result of this daring experiment – which we had to stop very quickly – was a kind of revelation. I had understood that when neocortex activity is eliminated, human beings have more similarities with other mammals: it facilitates childbirth. I understood the concept of neocortical inhibition and the solution that Nature has found to overcome the human handicap. The important point was to learn that the neocortex of a woman in labour must be at rest.

Since that time, we have learned a lot about the inhibitory effects of GHB and GABA.[6] In fact GHB has never held an important place in anaesthesiology. However, it has become associated with substance abuse and is thus a public health problem. Illegal forms are available under various names. The way that GHB reduces neocortical control means it has become a notorious 'date-rape drug' – in other words, it is used to facilitate sexual assault.

My understanding of the effects of neocortical inhibition during childbirth was later reactivated by other significant anecdotes. A young mother, in a two-bedroom ward, was celebrating the birth of her one-day-old baby. Her roommate was in pre-labour. Glasses of champagne were exchanged. The effect of the glass of champagne swallowed in one gulp by the roommate was so spectacular that the baby was born in a corridor after a real foetus ejection reflex. It is well known that champagne is a special wine. The bubbles immediately carry the alcohol to the brain. The power of alcohol to alter states of consciousness has been known since time immemorial. Today the mechanisms of action of alcohol are interpreted: one effect is to bind to GABA receptors.[7]

The ease with which schizophrenic women gave birth before modern antipsychotic treatments also helped me understand the physiological processes. Untreated schizophrenics do not have strong neocortical inhibitory abilities. We can also mention the cases of women in a vegetative coma who have given birth discreetly without the knowledge of those around them.

It is significant that psychedelic drugs known in terms of access to transcendence have also been used to facilitate childbirth. This is the case with cannabis, which has been, and still is, a sacred plant in many cultures. The biochemical effects of cannabinoids – the active substances in cannabis – have been well studied. In 1990, the discovery of cannabinoid receptors, in the brain in particular, and also of cannabinoids as neurotransmitters, suggested that cannabis acts as natural brain substances do. It has a well-known role in neocortical activity, with alterations in the perception of time and space.[6] The effects on the process of childbirth are therefore easy to interpret.

Daime, a drink whose generic name is ayahuasca, is another typical example of a drug used both to induce access to transcendence and also to facilitate the process of childbirth. It is the basis of a religious practice that began in the Amazon area and became a worldwide movement in the 1990s. Because the use of daime for religious purposes is legal in Brazil, some midwives are aware of its effects during childbirth and do not hesitate to share their observations.

When our capacity for long-term thinking is properly developed, when the concept of neocortical inhibition is assimilated, and when a prudent attitude towards substitute pharmacology is imposed, it will become inevitable that we seek out certain research paths. There is much to be learned, in particular, about the psychedelic substances produced by a wide variety of mushrooms. The current focus is on psilocybin. Of course, until now, the published studies have been in the field of psychiatry, with a particular interest in the treatment of depressive states. Understanding the physiology of childbirth as a chapter of brain physiology will be a necessary step toward the resurgence of shamanic midwifery.

It is likely that in the near future we will also have much to learn from psychoactive seaweeds, fish with psychedelic properties and hallucinogenic jellyfish. We'll probably rediscover what our ancestors who lived in coastal areas learned when the sea levels were significantly lower than they are today.

We must emphasise that we are referring to a one-off use of psychedelic drugs. We are outside the field of addiction. However, caution is called for due to the current state of our knowledge.

Beyond the simplistic scheme

We have chosen to remain inside the contrast between substitutive pharmacology and shamanic attitude. In fact, the distinction has been blurred at certain stages of history. Thus, in the middle of the 19th century there was a craze for the use of chloroform, after Queen Victoria gave birth to her eighth child after inhaling chloroform. It is difficult to classify this attitude. It is the same for the use of laughing gas (nitrous oxide), which combines a direct action on opiate receptors with an alteration of neocortical activity.

The history of 'twilight sleep' is significant. This expression is the quasi-official translation of the German word '*Dämmerschlaf*'. Twilight sleep, originally German, was a widely used method in the United States from the First World War until the advent of modern pharmacology. It is described as the combination of morphine, as a painkiller, and scopolamine, as an amnesic substance. It has been nearly forgotten that the German method originally combined pharmacology with sensory isolation that demonstrated a good understanding of physiological processes, even before the concept of neocortical inhibition was usable. The birthing rooms were dark and the uniforms were designed to minimise noise. In addition, women were sometimes blindfolded, and their ears were plugged with oil-soaked cotton. In other words, there were attempts to dissocialise childbirth. It is highly significant that only the pharmacological component of twilight sleep was taken into account and transmitted via the visitors.

The doula phenomenon

While contrasting the modern midwife as a technician trained to follow protocols and the shamanic midwife, we cannot help thinking of the mysterious doula phenomenon. Several memorable events have been instrumental in the development of my interest in this.

The first took place in February 1980, when Marshall Klaus visited us in the Pithiviers hospital (near Paris). He found it notable that six midwives, a group of help nurses, and I (as the only doctor) could cope with 1,000 births a year. He told me about the randomised controlled trial he was conducting in Guatemala with John Kennell (and others) about the presence of a female companion during birth. He was not yet using the term 'doula', which appeared in a September 1980 publication.[8] We shared our comments on this study, emphasising that it was useful in the context of the USA.

The second event took place in June 1998, when I was asked to do information sessions for doulas in London. I immediately noticed that most women participating in such sessions were radically different from those who had received an official European midwifery degree – almost always in their early twenties. These were mature women – most of them mothers or grandmothers – with a huge experience of life. I realised that, even in Europe, some pregnant women felt the need to rely on the same experienced mother-figure before, during, and after the birth. Liliana Lammers (who had had three homebirths in my presence) came to the first session. In December 2002, when she had acquired sufficient practical experience, we decided to cooperate and to complement each other in a renewed kind of information session. This was an opportunity to reconsider the dominant vocabulary. We eliminated the word 'training', which is too suggestive of an active role. We preceded the word 'doula' (which originally meant 'female slave') with the word 'paramana', a term that means 'next to the mother' and was acceptable to the Greek community (and those, like me, who had studied the Greek language).

The third event took place more than five hours east of Moscow by plane, in Krasnoyarsk, where I was invited to participate in the launching of the Siberian doula association in September 2013. Since that time, I have found it impossible to ignore that the doula phenomenon is global. When an unexpected phenomenon suddenly becomes global, two questions must be raised: 'What does it mean?' and 'What about the future?'

Until now the usual interpretations had subjective bases. Many pregnant women have expressed their feeling that current health systems – whether public or private, and whatever the country – cannot ideally satisfy their needs. At a time when the generation gap is deeper than ever, and in the age of nuclear or one-parent families, some women look for substitutes for their own mothers during the period surrounding birth.

This is precisely the phase of our history when a scientific language can easily describe the physiological continuity between the end of pregnancy, the birth process, and the interaction between mother and newborn baby.

After describing the physiological continuity between the end of pregnancy, birth, and the phase of interaction between mother and newborn baby, we are in a position to offer interpretations of the doula phenomenon. In terms of needs during the whole period surrounding birth, 'protection' remains the central concept. Since the mother is the prototype of the protective person, it appears only natural that some modern women feel the need to rely on the same mother figure before, during, and after giving birth.

What about the future of doulas?

Several scenarios are both possible and plausible.

In the most optimistic scenario, the doula phenomenon will be transitory, and will decline after successful participation in a paradigm shift. One can imagine that a new awareness will have the power to reverse the increasing tendency to classify the midwife as a highly specialised technician trained to follow protocols.[9] A renewed vocabulary, with the keyword 'protection', will be symptomatic of an actual new way of thinking.

However, according to the most pessimistic scenario, neither fast-developing branches of physiology nor the doula phenomenon will have the power to reverse thousands of years of conditioning. The dominant disempowering vocabulary will not radically evolve and will go on suggesting that during the period surrounding birth a woman needs the active participation of the cultural milieu: helping, guiding, controlling, coaching, managing, supporting, and so on. The term 'protection' will remain ignored.

Then the doula phenomenon will be a missed opportunity.

In the land of utopia... and elsewhere

We must realise that the current lack of understanding of birth physiology, as a chapter of brain physiology, goes hand in hand with a pharmacological assistance reduced to hormonal substitution. This analysis has led us to evoke, in a renewed scientific context, the possible resurgence and modernisation of an attitude whose primary objective is to facilitate certain physiological processes frequently inhibited by neocortical activity, instead of neutralising them and substituting for them. Does the shamanic midwife have a future... outside the land of utopia?[9]

6

Birth at home and birth elsewhere

The renewed horizon of bacteriologists
Since Pasteur's era, and until recently, there was a deep-rooted cultural conditioning associating microbes and diseases and classifying all microbes as enemies. This cultural conditioning was never seriously challenged while bacteriologists were only looking at microscopes and cultivating microbes on Petri dishes. However, the bacteriologists started to dramatically enlarge their horizons when they became geneticists, exploring the world of microorganisms by using the power of computer processing and new DNA sequencing technologies: not all bacteria seen under the microscope can be cultured, since their growth conditions are unknown. Bacteriologists can now see the 'unseen majority'.

In the age of the 'microbiome revolution', we must suddenly start from new bases to address the issue of birth environment. *Until recently, most women were giving birth in bacteriologically familiar and diversified environments. Today it is the opposite. One can claim that, from bacteriological (and therefore immunological) perspectives, the perinatal period is a phase of human life that has been radically altered in the past few decades.* Once more, it is a U-turn.

The human placenta
When raising questions inspired by this particularity of contemporary lifestyle, it suddenly appears essential to keep in mind that the types of placenta in different species

are classified according to the number of membranes separating the maternal and foetal blood circulation. Among mammals with epitheliochorial placentas (horses and pigs), with synepitheliochorial placentas (ruminants) and endotheliochorial placentas (carnivores), maternal antibodies are transferred via the colostrum.[1] Humans, higher primates and rodents have hemochorial placentas, with receptors for transfer of antibodies. In these species, maternal antibodies (namely IgG) are transferred to the foetus via the placenta. In humans, each of the four subclasses of IgG reach the foetus via active transport, which progressively increases in activity during pregnancy.[2-5] Foetal concentrations of IgG subclasses approximate to maternal concentrations at 38 weeks of pregnancy and continue to increase thereafter, occasionally reaching more than twice the maternal concentrations at the time of delivery. This is a specifically human trait, even among primates.[6,7]

The basic needs of the human neonate

The basic needs of neonates may be interpreted in the light of inter-species differences in placental structure and function. Among most mammals the priority is immediate access to colostrum: the early colostrum is, strictly speaking, vital. In humans, even if it is precious, early colostrum is not vital: *for thousands of years, the main effect of perinatal beliefs and rituals has been, more often than not, to deprive the neonate of early colostrum.* In our species, the main questions are about the bacteriological environment in the birthing place, how diverse it is and how familiar it is to the mother. Today, we are in a position to understand that the millions of microorganisms that will be the first to 'occupy the territory' will start programming the immune system. We must realise the importance of the topic, since it is about health development.

These considerations, inspired by immunology and

bacteriology, are instrumental in evaluating the scale of the recent turning point in the history of human births. A century ago, most women gave birth in a bacteriologically familiar environment. Today it is the opposite. There are of course degrees in how the bacteriological environment is altered in the perinatal period. Exposure to antibiotics and births by caesarean section in the sterile environment of an operating room are extreme examples.

On the day when a paradigm shift will push us to consider the perinatal period from these new perspectives, it will be impossible to skip new questions about the future of dysregulation of the immune system, particularly the prevalence of pathological conditions such as allergic diseases, auto-immune diseases and viral diseases. Up to now, epidemiological studies inspired by these questions have been exceptionally rare and have had to overcome technical difficulties, at a time when home birth is usually marginalised. It has been easier to contrast vaginal birth and caesarean birth inside the framework of conventional departments of obstetrics.

As a point of departure, we will need studies contrasting home births on the one hand and vaginal births in hospitals on the other. In practice, for multiple reasons, such studies are not feasible in emerging and wealthy countries, apart from the Netherlands. A Dutch birth cohort study involving more than 1,000 children (born at a time when the rate of home births was above 25% in that country) included data on birth characteristics, lifestyle factors, and allergic manifestations collected through repeated questionnaires from birth until age seven.[8] Faecal samples were collected at one month old to determine microbiota composition, and blood samples were collected at one, two and six to seven years to determine specific IgE levels. Home birth, compared with vaginal hospital birth, was associated with a decreased risk of atopic diseases and asthma. The differences were highly significant for children with atopic parents.

When the microbiome revolution is established, and when birth environment is widely studied from a bacteriological perspective, the development of new facets of the 'scientification of love' is probable. We'll focus on one example of a scientific topic of the future.

The function of kissing

In 1999, even in chapters entitled 'Sexual attractiveness' and 'The physiology of romantic love', it did not occur to me to raise questions about the function of kissing.[9] However, kissing appears as a universal behaviour among members of the chimpanzee family, including humans. There have been small preliminary studies, from hormonal perspectives, of mouth-to-mouth contact in the framework of genital sexuality. These studies evaluated in particular the levels of testosterone, oestrogens, dopamine and cortisol. It is difficult to look at oxytocin release, because oxytocin is the 'shy hormone' that does not easily appear in socialised environments. Kissing might be understood as an opportunity for a couple to activate and train in a synchronised way their oxytocin system, and to prepare for sexual intercourse.

Interestingly, there has been at least one valuable bacteriological study of 'French kissing'. Dutch researchers found that during an intimate kiss of 10 seconds there is an average total transfer of 80 million bacteria.[10] They investigated the effects of intimate kissing on the oral microbiota of 21 couples by self-administered questionnaires about their past kissing behaviour and by the evaluation of tongue and salivary microbiota samples in a controlled kissing experiment. In addition, they quantified the number of bacteria exchanged during intimate kissing by the use of marker bacteria introduced through the intake of a probiotic yoghurt drink by one of the partners prior to a second intimate kiss. Similarity indices of microbial communities show that average partners have a more similar oral microbiota composition compared to unrelated individuals, with by far the most pronounced similarity for communities associated with the tongue surface.

In the framework of the microbiome revolution, we are now expecting bacteriological studies of the function of kissing in the perinatal period. Since the advent of the socialisation of childbirth, the need many women feel to kiss their baby, when they are still in a specific physiologic state, has been repressed. This is a reason why it has been easier, until now, to study kissing behaviours in adults.

Meanwhile

The sudden new awareness induced by spectacular advances in bacteriology and immunology may already have practical implications. It is premature to transmit precise recipes. The point is to keep in mind that, ideally, the body of a newborn baby should be first colonised by a great diversity of familiar microbes.

We might mention typical examples of the possible immediate effects of this new awareness. Let us imagine the case of a home birth midwife who has understood, probably with the help of modern physiology, that 'protection' is the keyword associated with her role. Her main objective, until now, has been to protect the labouring woman against all situations that might induce adrenaline release or stimulate neocortical activity. Today, this midwife is in a position to realise that her role is also to protect the newborn baby against unfamiliar microbes. She will first think of how she might avoid transmitting too many of her own microbes. She will be worried by the presence in the house of unfamiliar human beings. On the other hand, she will not be worried by the family dog. The domestic dog is a carrier of familiar microbes. Furthermore, thanks to its powerful sense of smell, the dog can start identifying the newborn baby, and the odour of a human being is related to his (her) microbiome. So many new topics for scientific research!

For obvious reasons, the emergence of this new awareness cannot have the same effects in a hospital environment. From a bacteriological perspective, there is no substitute for home birth. However, some simple adaptive attitudes are possible, such as being more and more reluctant to expose foetuses and newborn babies to antibiotics. It is possible to give more importance to skin-to-skin contact immediately after birth and to rehabilitate kissing, even in the case of a caesarean section. It is also easy to wrap the baby in clothes recently worn by the mother and, occasionally, to put him or her in the arms of a person, such as the baby's father, who is cohabiting with the mother.

It is probable that several kinds of strategies will be evaluated in the near future. For example, the positive effects of the use of probiotics in the perinatal period need to be confirmed.[11] A pilot study in Puerto Rico has looked at the 'gauze-in-the vagina technique'.[12] A gauze pad is placed in the vagina in order to collect bacteria-laden secretions. Then, right after a caesarean birth, the neonate's skin and mouth are swabbed. This technique is based on the assumption that human babies have been programmed for immediate colonisation by vaginal microorganisms. There are good reasons to challenge this assumption. It is highly probable that birth with intact membranes ('birth in the caul') was frequent before the socialisation of childbirth. It is still comparatively common among modern women who give birth in an environment compatible with a 'foetus ejection reflex'.[13] It is notable that a great variety of societies have made the concordant observations that human beings born with the caul (i.e., protected against vaginal microbiota) will be healthy (and lucky).

To compensate the effects of microbial deprivation in the neonatal period, I have suggested the use of 'Bacille de

Calmette et Guerin' (BCG).[14,15] As a way to provide non-virulent microbes of the mycobacteria family, BCG is an immunomodulator previously used as a vaccine against tuberculosis and as a therapeutic agent in a great diversity of diseases. Theoretically, it should facilitate the kind of deviation of the immune system that is hindered in a more or less aseptic environment. It is the only vaccine used in infancy that has been evaluated through randomised controlled trials with long-term follow-up (in one study the follow up was 60 years!). It is notable that the long-term nonspecific effects on health always appeared to be positive. Trials with follow-up periods of less than 10 years would easily evaluate the prevalence of some of the dysregulations of the immune system that have become more frequent during the past decades.

Long-term thinking

There will probably come a time when it is impossible to ignore the bacteriological and immunological perspectives when addressing the issue of home birth versus hospital birth.

An effect of such a historical turning point should be to 'de-marginalise' home birth and therefore make it safer. It should be to raise questions about how to adapt home birth to the dominant urbanised lifestyle. Can a new awareness lead to a situation in which hospital staff will be at the service of an increased number of women who prefer to keep the option of home birth open? The prerequisite will be to overcome our deep-rooted cultural conditioning and to get out of the 'helping-guiding-controlling-supporting-coaching-managing paradigm'. It will be to understand the concept of 'protection of an involuntary process'. How long will it take us to truly accept that oxytocin is the 'shy hormone'?

7

Transformations of *Homo*

Examples of easily measurable transformations

Height is a valuable way to study transformations of *Homo* through prehistorical and historical time.

For example, it seems established that 40,000 years ago, European males such as Cro-Magnon were about 183cm tall. Yet 10,000 years ago, when our ancestors started to dominate Nature, European males were 162.5cm tall. Some 600 years ago male Europeans were around 165cm tall. Today they are 175cm tall. All these data stimulate curiosity and inspire countless theories. For example, there are reasons to wonder why young Dutch men are now averaging 183.8cm, after a short, spectacular, mysterious and unprecedented increase: they gained 20cm in the last 150 years. One of the most plausible interpretations is provided by the results of a 'Lifelines study' looking into the lives and health of more than 94,500 inhabitants in the northern parts of the Netherlands between 1935 and 1967.[1] It appears that the men with the greatest number of children were seven centimetres taller than average: they had 0.24 more children on average than the least fertile men, who were about 14cm below the average height.

Brain size is another measurable way to study the evolution of *Homo*. Around 100,000 years ago the average brain size was 1500cc. Today it is 1350cc.

Michel Odent

The future of the capacity to love

Many other transformations of *Homo* are already underway. Some of them cannot be ignored when considering the survival of our species. This is the case, in particular, of the oxytocin system, which is a spectacular example of a physiological function that has become suddenly less useful. It is becoming acceptable to claim that when physiological functions are underused, they become weaker from generation to generation. This is the case for the oxytocin system.

During the birth process, activation of the oxytocin system is supposed to reach another order of magnitude than during any other situation, even sexual intercourse and breastfeeding. At a time when the basic needs of labouring women need to be rediscovered, when synthetic oxytocin is cheap and widely used across the globe, and when the caesarean section has become an easy, fast and safe operation, the number of women who rely on their oxytocin system to give birth to babies and placentas is becoming insignificant. We must also keep in mind that a milk ejection reflex is induced by oxytocin release. After taking into account the current number of babies per woman and the short average duration of breastfeeding, it is easy to reckon that the number of milk ejection reflexes in the life of a modern woman is very small compared with what it has been in other societies: the oxytocin system is also underused to feed babies.

Should we expect that the probable transformations of *Homo* might include a weakening of the oxytocin system? I dare to go a step further and to suggest that perhaps this physiological system is already deteriorating. We can express concern about this possibility by bringing together a great diversity of published data. With regards to childbirth, let us just mention an American study called 'Changes in labor patterns over 50 years'.[2] The authors compared a first group of nearly 40,000 births that occurred between 1959 and 1966 and a second group of nearly 100,000 births that occurred between 2002 and 2008. They only looked at births of one baby at term, with head presentation and spontaneous initiation of labour. After taking into account many factors such as the age, height and weight of the mother, it appeared that the duration of the first stage of labour was dramatically longer in the second group. It was two and a half hours longer in the case of a first baby, and two hours in the other cases. For practitioners of my generation this study demonstrates the obvious: before being aware of such data, I was already personally convinced that the human capacity to give birth is deteriorating.

We might also mention countless studies suggesting that in spite of intense public health campaigns to promote breastfeeding, and although contemporary populations are better informed than ever about the irreplaceable value of mother's milk, recent statistics about breastfeeding are worrying. As for genital sexuality, many factors are involved and hard data are not available, but one can observe that most sex therapists are overworked and that drugs to correct sexual dysfunctions are at the top of the lists of pharmaceutical substances in terms of commercial value.

The future of the capacity to love appears to be a serious topic at a time when it is well accepted that the oxytocin system is involved in all facets of love. The capacity for empathy, as a facet of love, is a personality trait that has been evaluated through scores developed by modern psychological sciences. At the annual meeting of the Association for Psychological Science in June 2010, a synthesis of 72 studies of the evolution of personality traits of American students (college graduates) between 1979 and 2009 was presented.[3] According to this research, college graduates are 40% less empathetic than those of twenty to thirty years ago. The decline has been progressive, particularly after the year 2000. Once more, this is compatible with a declining oxytocin system.

While it appears unrealistic, perhaps even impossible, to re-establish the laws of natural selection in humans, we can still wonder whether there are possible ways to interfere. What can we do so that oxytocin – as the main component of all cocktails of 'love hormones' – has opportunities to be intensely released as early as possible during human life? Would it be possible, for example, to direct the dominant conditioning? Would it be possible to spread the word and convince anyone that, in terms of reproductive physiology, human beings are mature before the age of 20? In other words, can we underline the advantages of having a first baby around the age of 18? What would be the effects of combining such considerations with a renewed understanding of birth physiology?

8

Can humanity survive socialised access to transcendence?

We have presented the socialisation of childbirth as a crucial facet of the domination of Nature that started with the 'Neolithic revolution' about 10,000 years ago. We have also provided reasons to present an authentic 'foetus ejection reflex' as a 'highway to transcendence'. The time has come to mix the issues of human birth and emotional states giving access to another reality than space and time: they are indissociable in an emergent scientific context.

Inherent in human nature?

The first step is to recall that in human groups with a Palaeolithic lifestyle, women used to isolate themselves to give birth: 'privacy' was undoubtedly their basic need.[1-3] The second step is to convince anyone that our Palaeolithic ancestors undoubtedly had access to transcendence. One simple way is to mention what we know about Venus figurines.

Most figurines have been unearthed in Europe, but others have been found as far away as Siberia, and distributed across much of Eurasia. They have been dated to different phases of the Paleolithic era. Most of them exaggerate the abdomen, hips, breasts, thighs, or vulva. The most plausible interpretation is that a Venus figurine is an archetype of a female Supreme Creator. There are other reasons to be convinced that access to transcendence is universal among large-brained *Homo*. Thus, after studying sites of ceremonial activity, researchers believe they have detected the expression of access to transcendence more than 400,000 years ago in places such as the cave of Denisova in southern Siberia and the Qesem caves in Israel.[4]

Today we are in a position to claim that transcendent emotional states are inherent in human nature and that they became socialised at the same time as childbirth.

Culturally acceptable pathways

Since the Palaeolithic period, all societies have developed and promoted pathways to transcendence that were considered culturally acceptable. For example, prayer, fasting, music, singing, and psychedelic herbs can be controlled pathways. From the time when access to transcendence was not considered a private event, specialised buildings became essential in all villages, towns and cities: temples, churches, cathedrals, mosques, synagogues and so on.

Modern scientific research is influenced by dominant, deeply rooted conditioning: in general, deliberately human-induced states of consciousness are the most studied. Ecstatic/orgasmic states related to reproduction are not easily accepted topics in academic circles. They are often associated with negative connotations.

A vocabulary analysis is an eloquent way to realize that the *organs and physiological functions directly involved in human reproduction are associated with the concept of shame*. In English, for example, 'pudendal' is used in scientific language to refer to the genitals, which are innervated by the 'pudendal nerves' and receive their blood through the 'pudendal arteries'. The root of these words is the Latin verb *'pudere'*, which means 'to be ashamed'.

The same is true in a wide variety of languages. In French, the term *'honte'* is used: *'nerfs honteux', 'arteres honteuses'*, and so on. In Chinese, the pubic bone is called *'Chigu'*, which literally means 'bone of shame'. In Japanese, the penis is often called 'the son', suggesting that using a specific or overly explicit term would be a violation of cultural norms that would induce a sense of shame.

It is as if, for thousands of years, many aspects of human nature have been concealed by deep-rooted conditioning. In a renewed scientific context, we cannot ignore that certain physiological functions, which have been commonly altered for ages, are potentially associated with ecstatic states. This is how I introduced the concept of 'highways to transcendence' when referring to episodes of human reproductive life such as the 'foetus ejection reflex', the 'milk ejection reflex' and the 'sperm ejection reflex'. All these events have similarities that may be studied in the context of physiological states associated with reduced neocortical control facilitating specific hormonal balances. Without multiplying the anecdotes, I will simply point out that the rare modern women who have given birth with an authentic foetus ejection reflex and who were in an ecstatic state at the moment of their very first contact with the newborn, claim to have been transformed by this experience. This is the prototype of an emotional state that is not studied by modern science.

There are obvious reasons why scientific studies of transcendent emotional states must overcome specific difficulties. One of the main reasons is that access to transcendence can occur at any age and in a great diversity of circumstances.

As a general rule it appears that the capacity to experience transcendent emotional states is comparatively weak in mid-adulthood, when neocortical inhibitions are as powerful as possible. However, this capacity can emerge occasionally, in particular during ecstatic/orgasmic states related to reproductive functions.

Furthermore, there are individual particularities related

to personality traits. For example, an inverse correlation has been found between personality traits associated with high density of available serotonin receptors and scores of transcendence.[5] As a general rule, efficient neocortical control has inhibitory effects: 'Blessed are the poor in spirit, for theirs is the Kingdom of Heaven' (Matthew 5:3).

We must keep in mind that specific pathological conditions could also be classified as 'highways to transcendence'. This is the case of Geschwind's syndrome in the context of temporal lobe epilepsy.[6] This syndrome includes easy access to transcendent emotional states. It appears to be related to a particular connectivity between the temporal neocortex and primitive brain structures.[7] Although it is difficult, in retrospect, to establish firm and uncontested diagnoses, it has been claimed that many well-known mystics had conditions compatible with temporal lobe epilepsy. It has been reported, for example, that during his conversion on the road to Damascus, St Paul was blind for three days, fell to the ground and had ecstatic visions. Muhammad described falling episodes accompanied by visual and auditory hallucinations. Joseph Smith, who founded Mormonism, reported blackouts and speech interruptions, and once found himself lying on the ground. As for Joan of Arc, a great light accompanied the voice she heard. In our cultural milieus, the study of mental health is an acceptable way to try to interpret the routes to transcendence.

There are reasons to claim that elderly human beings, whose neocortical activity is weakening, may have an increased capacity to experience transcendent emotional states. This remains within the realm of empirical knowledge, although a new generation of studies might investigate this topic further.[8] It is significant that Lars Tornstam, from Uppsala University, could create the 'Gerotranscendence Scale', while studying access to transcendence in the particular case of elderly people.[9]

It has also long been understood that access to transcendence is particularly easy in childhood, when the neocortex is not yet mature: 'Suffer the little children to come unto me' (Mark 10:14). It is significant that catechisms are used, in particular, for the education of children, at an age when they are highly receptive, before the critical phase of adolescence.

Learning from Pascal

On Monday 23 November 1654, when Pascal was 31 years old, he had, before midnight, a mystical crisis that lasted more than two hours. There was no witness. Pascal never spoke about this, not even with his close relatives and friends, such as his two sisters, the Duke of Rouannez, Father Beurrier and Antoine Singlin, his director at Port-Royal. We would never have heard about this episode except that eight years later, a few days after Pascal's death, a servant noticed by chance that in the inner pocket of the deceased's jacket there was something which seemed thicker than the rest. He peeled it off to see what it was. He found two copies of a kind of memorial which Pascal had written secretly after what he obviously considered a private key event in his life.[10] From that time on, Pascal had felt the need to publicly contrast two realities: 'Reason' – providing exclusive access to space and time reality – and 'Heart'. During his mystical experience, he had access to 'God' and 'Jesus', terms that were at his disposal in the context of the 17th century. His attitude was a significant way to confirm that access to transcendence, whatever the context, is a solitary experience. Several centuries before the advent of modern neurophysiology, its concepts and its vocabulary, the genial polymath Pascal, as author of Les Pensées, was in a position to consider what we can now call neocortical control and neocortical inhibition as keys to understanding human nature and, in particular, access to transcendence.

Today, we must raise questions about the future, at the very time when some aspects of Pascal's work are suddenly more topical than ever before. Let us first emphasise that *the current obvious decline of the capacity to give birth is concomitant with the decline of the capacity to have access to transcendence.*

9

In the beginning was the word

At a time when the limits of the domination of Nature have suddenly been reached, human adaptability is put to the test. Until now, human adaptability has been considered almost limitless, when taking into account criteria such as adaptation to latitude, altitude, nutrition, coastal and inland areas and so on. Today, in order to survive, human beings must radically and urgently adapt to new ways of thinking. This implies the need for a new vocabulary.

Paradigm shift

I suggest the modern phrase 'paradigm shift' as symbolic of the current crisis. How and to what extent can modern *Homo* initiate a new way of thinking? Until now, this facet of human adaptability has not been seriously considered. However, we can learn through anecdotes that there are significant individual differences and that the way of thinking is age dependent.

As knowledge, and indirectly ways of thinking, has been mostly transmitted through written language, there has been a tendency, among experts, to select – as publishable – documents that provide information without altering the dominant way of thinking. There have always been subtle mechanisms of protection against paradigm shift. This is at the root of what we call today the 'peer review process'.

I do not hesitate to present the New Testament as the prototype of peer-reviewed documents. There are four

Gospels that were selected for publication by authoritative experts. Other gospels did not make it through the selection process: they disappeared, or survived in a clandestine way. The proto-gospel of James was saved from oblivion in the middle of the 19th century by the Austrian mystic Jacob Lorber.[1] This is why we can now compare the reports of the birth of Jesus by Luke and James.

According to Luke, the birth was quite conventional. The travellers urgently stopped in an improvised available place; Mary wrapped her son in swaddling clothes and laid him in a manger. This scene was publishable in a peer-reviewed document.

It is another matter if we refer to the report by James. Joseph had found a midwife. When the midwife and Joseph entered the improvised birthing place, Jesus had already been born. It was only when a dazzling light had faded that the midwife realized she was facing an incredible scene: Jesus had already found his mother's breast! Then the midwife said: *'Who has ever seen a barely born baby taking his mother's breast? This is an obvious sign that when he becomes a man, this child will judge the world according to Love and not according to the Law!'*

The scene was so unrealistic that it was not taken seriously. What if the report of James had not been censored by the peer-review process? Our duty is to interpret and to evaluate the paramount importance of the reaction of the midwife, and to realise that there was a missed opportunity in the history of the domination of Nature.

Today, about two millennia after the publication of the Gospels, we are inundated by peer-reviewed documents. We are in the age of 'circular epidemiology'. This means that similar studies are constantly repeated, even if the results are known in advance. To emphasise the frequent negative side-effects of the current publication process, I tried to use a term that would be the opposite of 'circular epidemiology'.

This is how I introduced the concept of 'cul-de-sac epidemiology'.[2] The results of studies in this framework are shunned by the medical community and the media. 'Cul-de-sac epidemiological studies' are not replicated, even by the original investigators, and are rarely quoted after publication. They disturb most peer reviewers because they imply new ways of thinking.

I offer the example of a Swedish study, published in 1990 by Bertil Jacobson, leading to the conclusion that certain obstetric drugs (opiates, laughing gas) are risk factors for drug addiction in adult offspring.[3] The results have never been confirmed or invalidated by further research. Yet drug addiction is one of the main preoccupations of our time.

In spite of the many reasons for pessimism, there are reasons for optimism. The main one is provided by anecdotes of influential people who have radically changed their way of thinking within a short period. The case of Frederick Leboyer is an eloquent example.

From Leboyer I to Leboyer II

In 1974, Leboyer had awakened us with the bestseller *Pour une naissance sans violence* (*Birth Without Violence*).[4] From this work of art (and the film that complemented it), many have remembered above all the bath given to the newborn by someone such as the doctor. In the maternity unit of the French hospital where I was practising at that time, when a baby was born, there was usually a woman on duty who had read Leboyer and was eager to experience the pleasure of bathing the newborn. This significant scene helped to reinforce my interest in the relationship between human beings and water.

In order to understand the revolutionary dimension of the words of 'Leboyer 1974', it is necessary to recall the historical context. Until then, we were almost exclusively interested in how women were giving birth. Suddenly, through a book inspired by a therapy that allowed him to 'reexperience his birth', Leboyer spoke on behalf of newborn babies. In answer to the question 'which hands should hold the child?' he wrote that many modern mothers 'have still, lifeless, uncomprehending hands'. The baby must first be 'held by hands that know'.

In 1982, in a little-known masterpiece published in French only, Fréderick Leboyer, as a talented poet, dared to write:

L'intimité, c'est deux.
Trois, c'est déjà la collectivité, sa brutalité, sa grossièreté.
Aussi bien, la mère et son nouveau-né ... ces amants,
Comment se connaitraient-ils, se reconnaitraient-ils
Autrement que seul à seul, dans l'ombre complice?[5]

This is an unofficial translation:

Intimacy always two
Three already a crowd... brutal, rude
A mother and her newborn baby... these lovers
How can they recognise each other, if not
one to one, in a complicit shade?

How, within a few years, did we go from one Leboyer to the other? How can we interpret such a spectacular mutation? The first reason is that, in a rapidly changing scientific context, it suddenly became possible to go deeper into the concept of 'hands that know'. To do this, we must first understand the solution that nature found to make human births possible. Despite millennia of socialisation of the period surrounding birth, some women find the power to give birth by themselves if they cut themselves off from the world by putting at rest their powerful 'new brain' (the neocortex) that radically distinguishes human beings from all other mammals.

As soon as he or she are born, the baby is in the hands of an 'instinctive' mother who knows how to hold them. She feels the need to touch her baby, to smell their smell, to meet their eyes… if she is not distracted. Thus, she does not come back brutally 'to our planet'. She can release the hormonal flow that facilitates the delivery of the placenta. It is vital. The baby, on the other hand, expresses the need to identify the mother. A primitive sensory function such as smell plays an essential role between two human mammals whose behaviour is barely under neocortical control. It is no longer possible to separate the study of maternal and neonatal physiological functions. It becomes difficult to separate the newborn from the mother, when the key word is 'interaction'.

Let's also keep in mind that shortly after birth, the newborn, if not distracted, behaves as if he or she is looking for the nipple. This is the rooting reflex. The mother, if she has given birth by herself, knows how to adapt to what seems to be a demand. Thus, after thousands of years of beliefs and rituals that postponed the initiation of breastfeeding, we have learned that human beings seem to have been programmed to find the breast without any delay.[6]

We can now conclude by presenting the hour after birth as the worst possible time to give a child a bath.

Frédérick Leboyer deserves our gratitude. It is a feat to do such a U-turn in a few years.

Let us open together the doors of a new paradigm

Addendum

Childbirth in the land of Utopia

January 2031

As everybody knows, our country – Utopia – is an independent territory.

In spite of our high scientific and technological level, we have maintained and even developed our main cultural characteristics. We have developed in particular our capacity to make unrealistic projects and to smash the limits of political correctness. We shall illustrate the specificity of the Utopian culture by referring to the history of childbirth.

In 2010 two local celebrities had chosen to give birth by caesarean. This is how childbirth became suddenly one of the main topics for discussion in the media. We all realised that every year the rate of caesareans was higher than the year before. The dominant opinion was in favour of authoritarian guidelines by the Utopian Health Organisation (UHO). To face such an unprecedented situation the Head of UHO decided to organise a multidisciplinary meeting.

A statistician spoke first. He presented impressive graphs, starting in 1950, when the low segmental technique of caesarean replaced the classical technique. According to his extrapolations it was highly probable that after 2020 the caesarean would be a common way to give birth. A well-known obstetrician felt obliged to immediately comment on this data. He claimed that we should look at the positive aspect of this new phenomenon. He explained how the caesarean had become an easy, fast and safe operation. He was convinced that in the near future most women would prefer to avoid the risks associated with a delivery by the vaginal route. To support his point of view about the safety of the caesarean, he presented a Canadian series, published in 2007, of more than 46,000 elective caesareans for breech presentation at 39 weeks with zero maternal death, and an American series, published in 2009, of 24,000 repeated caesareans with one neonatal death. He explained that in many situations an elective pre-labour caesarean was by far the safest way to have a baby. He concluded that 'we cannot stop progress'. While he was speaking it was clear from her body language that a midwife at the meeting thought that there was something the doctor had not understood.

A very articulate lady, the president of ABWL ('Association for Birth With Love') immediately reacted to the conclusion by the doctor. She first asked him which criteria he was using to evaluate the safety of the caesarean. Of course he mentioned perinatal mortality/morbidity rates and maternal mortality/morbidity rates. Then the president of ABWL explained that this limited list of criteria had been established long ago, before the 21st century, and that a great diversity of developing scientific disciplines now suggested a list of new criteria to evaluate the practices of obstetrics and midwifery. This was the turning point of this historical multidisciplinary meeting.

The Professor of Hormonology immediately echoed this eloquent and convincing comment. After referring to an accumulation of data regarding the behavioural effects of hormones involved in childbirth, he could easily conclude that to have babies women had been programmed to release a real 'cocktail of love hormones'. During the hour following birth, he explained clearly, maternal and foetal hormones released during the birth process are not yet eliminated and each of them has a specific role to play in the interaction between mother and neonate. In other words, he added, thanks to the hormonal perspective we can now interpret the concept of critical periods introduced by behavioural scientists: some pioneers in this field had understood, as early as in the middle of the 20th century, that among all mammals there is, immediately after birth, a short period of time that will never happen again and that is critical in mother-baby attachment. He dared to conclude that by combining the data he had provided with the results of countless epidemiological studies suggesting that the way we are born has life-long consequences, it was becoming clear that the capacity to love develops to a great extent in the perinatal period. The obstetrician was gaping at him.

After such conclusions by the Professor of Hormonology, the head of the department of epidemiology of UHO could not remain silent. This epidemiologist had a special interest in 'primal health research'. He had collected hundreds of published studies detecting risk factors in the perinatal period for a great diversity of pathological conditions in adulthood, adolescence or childhood. He offered an overview of the most valuable studies, particularly those involving huge numbers of subjects. He summarised the results of his enquiries by noticing that when researchers study pathological conditions that can be interpreted as different sorts of impaired capacity to love (to love others or to love oneself) from a primal health research perspective, they always detect risk factors in the perinatal period. Referring to the comments by the president of ABWL about the need for new criteria to evaluate the practices of obstetrics and midwifery, he emphasised the need to think long term. Finally, he presented the Primal Health Research Databank as a tool to train ourselves to think long term.

Then a geneticist impatiently raised her hand. She presented the concept of 'gene expression' as another way to interpret the life-long consequences of pre- and perinatal events. She explained that among the genetic material human beings receive at conception, some genes will become silent without disappearing. The gene expression phenomenon is influenced in particular by environmental factors during the pre- and perinatal periods. The obstetrician was more and more attentive and curious, as if discovering a new topic. One of his judicious questions about the genesis of pathological conditions and personality traits gave the geneticist the opportunity to explain that the nature of an environmental factor is often less important than the time of the interaction. She explained the concept of a critical period for gene-environment interaction. The presentation by the geneticist induced a fruitful interdisciplinary conversation. The epidemiologist jumped on a question by a general practitioner to provide more details about one of the new functions of the Primal Health Research Database, which is to give some clues about the critical period for gene-environment interaction regarding different pathological conditions or personality traits.

A bacteriologist, who had kept a low profile since the beginning of the session, emphasised that the minutes following birth are critical from his perspective as well. Few people had previously understood that at the very time of birth the newborn baby is germ free and that some hours later millions of microbes will have colonised their body. Because the antibodies called IgG easily cross the human placenta he explained that the microbes familiar for the mother are already familiar for the germ-free newborn baby, and therefore friendly. He commented that when babies are born via the perineum, it is guaranteed that they are first contaminated by a multitude of germ satellites of the mother, compared with babies born by caesarean. He contrasted birth at home and birth elsewhere. In order to stress the importance of the question, he mentioned that our gut flora is to a great extent established during the minutes following birth: useful considerations at a time when we are learning that this intestinal flora represents 80% of our immune system.

The bacteriologist agreed when a baby feeding adviser added that, in the right environment, if mother and newborn baby are not separated at all, there is a high probability that the baby will find the breast during the hour following birth and will consume the early colostrum with its friendly germs, specific local antibodies and anti-infectious substances. The consumption of early colostrum probably has long-term consequences, at least by influencing the way the gut flora is established.

The head of UHO was obviously happy with the progress of the interdisciplinary meeting he had organised. He asked an old philosopher, considered the wise man of the community, to conclude. The philosopher explained that we should not ignore a specifically human dimension and that we must first and foremost think in terms of civilisation. He referred to the data provided by the epidemiologist. Among the studies he presented huge numbers had often been necessary to detect tendencies and statistically significant effects. This was a way to keep in mind that where human beings are concerned, we must often forget individuals, anecdotes and particular cases, and reach the collective and therefore cultural dimension. From what had been heard during this meeting, it was clear that humanity was in an unprecedented situation that he summarised in a very concise way. Today, he said, the number of women who give birth to babies and placentas thanks to the release of what is a real cocktail of love hormones is approaching zero. What will happen in terms of civilisation if we go on that way? What will happen after two or three generations if love hormones are made useless during the critical period surrounding birth?

After such an eloquent conclusion the head of the UHO asked the participants their point of view about the need to control the rate of caesarean. Everybody, including the

obstetrician, found the need for action necessary, even urgent.
This is how a second meeting was planned in order to find effective solutions.

At the beginning of the second meeting the head of UHO asked the participants if they had solutions to suggest in order to control the rate of caesarean and other obstetrical interventions. The obstetrician presented a project 'to assess the effectiveness of a multifaceted strategy for improving the appropriateness of indications for caesarean'. Nobody paid attention. A recently graduated young doctor spoke about the need to reconsider the education of medical and midwifery students. The head of the midwifery school immediately replied that all over the world there have been many attempts to re-adapt the education of midwives and doctors, including specialised doctors, without any significant positive effects on birth outcomes. Several participants spoke about financial incentives to moderate the rates of obstetrical intervention. The head of UHO intervened and stressed that this solution had been unsuccessfully tried in several countries and that caesarean rates were increasing in all countries whatever the health system: we should therefore look at other factors. He added that the risk would be to increase the incidence of long and difficult births by the vaginal route with an overuse of pharmacological substitutes for natural hormones. This effect would be unacceptable at a time when caesarean had become such an easy and fast operation. The priority should be to try first to make births as easy as possible in order to reduce the need for obstetrical interventions in general.

Unexpectedly, the turning point in the discussion occurred when a neurophysiologist – internationally known for her studies of the behaviour of *mantis religiosa*, a variety of praying mantis – intervened for the first time. She explained that by

Michel Odent

mixing her scientific studies and her experience as a mother, she had acquired a clear understanding of the basic needs of labouring women. In general, she said, the messages sent by the central nervous system to the genitalia are inhibitory. She understood this simple rule when studying the mating behaviour of *mantis religiosa*. During sexual intercourse in this species the female often eats the head of the male; a radical way to eliminate inhibitory messages! Then the sexual activity of the male is dramatically reinforced and the chance of conception is increased. She had understood that the inhibitory effect of the central nervous system on all episodes of sexual life is a general rule. She had many opportunities to confirm this rule and, interestingly, she understood it still more clearly after giving birth to her first baby. She was convinced that the reduction in neocortical activity was the main reason why her birth was so easy and fast. She recalled that human beings are characterised by the enormous development of the part of the central nervous system called the neocortex. Her neocortex was obviously at complete rest when she was in established labour since she had completely forgotten many details about the place where she gave birth. She remembered vaguely that she was in a rather dark place, and that there was nobody around but a midwife sitting in a corner and knitting. She also remembered that at a certain phase of labour she was vomiting and the midwife just said: 'this happened to me when I had my second baby: it's normal'. Although imprecise in her memory, she was convinced that this discreet comment, in a whispering motherly voice, had facilitated the progress of labour. With this experienced and calm mother figure she could feel perfectly secure. In retrospect, all the conditions were met to reduce the activity of her neocortex. She could feel secure without feeling observed, in semi-darkness and silence. So, her practical suggestion, after combining what she had learned as a neurophysiologist and what she had learned as a mother, was to reconsider the criteria used to select the midwifery students. The prerequisite to enter a midwifery school of the future would be to have had personal experience of giving birth without any medical intervention, and to consider this birth a positive experience.

The obstetrician was not comfortable with this suggestion, claiming that he had been working with wonderful midwives who were not mothers. The head of the midwifery school retorted that everybody knows good midwives who are not mothers. However, her duty was to offer the guarantee that the midwives graduating from her school share personality traits that mean that their presence close to a birthing woman would disturb the progress of labour as little as possible. This is why she could not imagine better criteria than those suggested by the neurophysiologist. Because this suggestion was outside the usual limits of political correctness, it was immediately considered by almost everybody as acceptable in the land of Utopia.

Then a male voice was heard from a corner of the room. It was the voice of the young technician whose role was to record the session: 'As an outsider, can I ask a naïve question? What if the prerequisite to be qualified as an obstetrician was also to have had a personal experience of giving birth without any medical intervention and to consider this birth as a positive experience?'

At this, it was as if everybody in the room was in the situation of Archimedes shouting 'Eureka!'...an unforgettable collective enthusiasm! It was immediately obvious to all the participants that such a project was unrealistic enough to be adopted without any further discussion and without any delay in the land of Utopia.

A committee was immediately set up, in order to organise a 15-year period of transition.

Today, in January 2031, we can offer valuable statistics, since the period of transition ended in 2024. These statistics are impressive.

Perinatal mortality rates are as low as in all countries with similar standards of living. The rate of transfer to paediatric units has dramatically decreased. There has not been a single case of forceps delivery for four years. Since the priority is to avoid long and difficult labours by the vaginal route, the use of ventouse and the use of drugs are exceptionally rare. However, the rates of caesarean are three times lower than before the period of transition. A paedopsychiatrist has already mentioned that autism is less common than in the past. If the respected philosopher – the wise man of the community – was still alive, he would state that now, in the land of Utopia, most women give birth to babies and placentas thanks to the release of a 'cocktail of love hormones'.

The new head of UHO and his teams are preparing articles for different sorts of international media. They have launched a 'call for five-word slogans' in order to urgently spread the word in a concise and effective way. This is the selected slogan:

ONLY UTOPIA CAN SAVE HUMANITY!

About the author

Michel Odent MD was in charge of the surgical unit and the maternity unit at the Pithiviers (France) state hospital from 1962–85.

For many years he was the only doctor overseeing around 1,000 births a year. He is the author of the first article in the medical literature about the initiation of lactation during the hour following birth (1977), the first article about the use of birthing pools (1983), and the first article applying the 'gate control theory of pain' to obstetrics (1975).

He created the Primal Health Research database (www.primalhealthresearch.com) and he has been a member of the Professional Advisory Board of La Leche League International for 40 years. He is a Visiting Professor at the Odessa National Medical University and Doctor Honoris Causa of the University of Brasilia.

Many of his previous books are also published by Pinter & Martin.

References

Chapter One: Spectacular U-turns
1. Eaton, S.B., Shostak, M., Konner, M. *The paleolithic prescription*, Harper and Row, New York, 1988.
2. Wulf Schiefenhovel, 'Childbirth among the Eipos, New Guinea'. Film presented at the Congress of Ethnomedicine, 1978, Gottingen, Germany.
3. Daniel Everett, *Don't sleep, there are snakes*, Profile Books, 2008.
4. Jacques Gelis, *L'Arbre et le Fruit*, Fayard, Paris, 1984.
5. Nordtveit, T.I., Melve, K.K., et al. 'Maternal and paternal contribution to intergenerational recurrence of breech delivery: population-based cohort study'. *BMJ* 2008 Apr 19;336 (7649):872-6. doi: 10.1136.
6. Vázquez-Calzada, J.L. 'Cesarean childbirth in Puerto Rico: the facts', *Health Sci J.* 1997 Dec; 16(4):395-400.

Chapter Two: A U-turn in our understanding of human nature
1. https://www.science.org/content/article/bonobos-join-chimps-closest-human-relatives
2. Jenkins, D.T., Wysocki, S.J., Davies, D.M. 'Amniotic fluid squalene: A useful test in prolonged pregnancy', *Aust N Z J Obstet Gynaecol* 1982; 22: 135-7
3. Pickens, W.L., Warner, R.R., et al. 'Characterization of vernix caseosa: water content, morphology, and elemental analysis', *Journal of Investigative Dermatology* 2000;115 (5): 875-881.
4. Wang, D.H., Ran-Ressler, R., et al. 'Sea Lions develop Human-like Vernix Caseoa delivering branched fats and squalene to the GI tract'. *Sci Rep* 2018; 8(1):7478. doi: 10.1038/s41598-018-25871-1.PMID: 29748625
5. Guess, K., Malek, L., Anderson, A., et al. 'Knowledge and practices regarding iodine supplementation: A national survey of healthcare providers'. *Women Birth* 2016 Sep 2. pii: S1871-

5192(16)30094-4. doi: 10.1016/j.wombi.2016.08.007. [Epub ahead of print]

6. Plourde, M., Cunnane, S.C. 'Extremely limited synthesis of long-chain polyunsaturates in adults: implications for their dietary essentiality and use as supplements'. *Appl Physiol Nutr Metab* 2007; 32(4):619-34

7. Burdge, G.C., Wootton, S.A. 'Conversion of alpha-linolenic acid to eicosapentaenoic, docosapentaenoic and docosahexaenoic acids in young women'. *Br J Nutr*, 88 (2002), pp. 411-420

8. Burdge, G.C., Jones, A.E., Wootton, S.A. 'Eicosapentaenoic and docosapentaenoic acids are the principal products of a-linolenic acid metabolism in young men'. *British Journal of Nutrition* (2002), 88, 355–363.

9. Young, S.M., Benyshek, D.C. 'In search of human placentophagy: a cross-cultural survey of human placenta consumption, disposal practices, and cultural beliefs'. *Ecology of Food and Nutrition* 2010; 49: issue 6. Pages 467-484.

10. Odent, Michel 'Obstetrical implications of waterside hypothesis', *Journal of Prenatal and Perinatal Psychology & Health* 2012; 26 (3).

11. Kristal, M.B. 'Enhancement of opioid-mediated analgesia: A solution to the enigma of placentophagia'. *Neuroscience & Biobehavioral Reviews* 1991; 15 (3): 425-435

12. Davis, R.W., Pierotti, V.R., et al. 'Lipoproteins in pinnipeds: analysis of a high molecular weight form of apolipoprotein E'. *Journal of Lipid Research* 1991; 32(6):1013-23.

13. Boule, M. (1911–1913) *L'Homme fossile de La Chapelle-aux-Saints* [The Fossil Man from La Chapelle-aux-Saints] Masson, Paris.

14. Trinkaus, E., Samsel, M., Villotte, S. 'External auditory exostoses among western Eurasian late Middle and Late Pleistocene humans'. *PLoS One*. 2019 Aug 14;14(8): e0220464.

15. Simas, V., Hing, W., Furness, J., et al. The Prevalence and Severity of External Auditory Exostosis in Young to

Quadragenarian-Aged Warm-Water Surfers. *Sports* 2020, *8*(2), 17; https://doi.org/10.3390/sports8020017

16. Smith-Guzmán, N.E., Cooke, R.G. 'Cold-water diving in the tropics? External auditory exostoses among the Pre-Columbian inhabitants of Panama', *American Journal of Physical Anthropology* 2019 Mar;168(3):448-458. doi: 10.1002/ajpa.23757. Epub 2018 Dec 21

17. Rhys Evans, P.H., Cameron, M. 'Aural exostoses (surfer's ear) provide vital fossil evidence of an aquatic phase in Man's early evolution', *Ann R Coll Surg Engl* 2017 Nov; 99(8):594-601. doi: 10.1308/rcsann.2017.0162. Epub 2017 Sep

Chapter Three: 'If you consume the fruit of the tree of knowledge... in sorrow you'll give birth'

1. Endevelt-Shapira, Y., Shushan, S., Roth, Y., Sobel, N. 'Disinhibition of olfaction: human olfactory performance improves following low levels of alcohol'. *Behav Brain Res.* 2014 Oct 1;272:66-74. doi: 10.1016/j.bbr.2014.06.024. Epub 2014 Jun 25.

2. Odent, M. 'The early expression of the rooting reflex'. Proceedings of the 5th International Congress of Psychosomatic Obstetrics and Gynaecology, Rome 1977. London: Academic Press, 1977: 1117-19.

3. Odent, M. '*L'expression précoce du réflexe de fouissement*'. In: *Les cahiers du nouveau-né*. Paris 1978; 1-2: 169-185.

4. Marlier, L., Schaal, B., Soussignan, R. 'Orientation responses to biological odours in the human newborn. Initial pattern and postnatal plasticity'. *C R Acad Sci III.* 1997 Dec;320(12):999-1005. PMID: 9587477 [PubMed - indexed for MEDLINE]

5. Varendi, H., Porter, R.H., Winberg, J. 'The effect of labor on olfactory exposure learning within the first postnatal hour'. *Behav Neurosci.* 2002 Apr;116(2):206-11. PMID: 11996306 [PubMed - indexed for MEDLINE]

6. Cernoch, J.M., Porter, R.H. 'Recognition of maternal axillary

odors by infants'. *Child Dev.* 1985 Dec;56(6):1593-8.
7. Sullivan, R.M., Toubas, P. 'Clinical usefulness of maternal odor in newborns: soothing and feeding preparatory responses'. *Biol Neonate.* 1998 Dec;74(6):402-8.
8. Varendi, H., Christensson, K., Porter, R.H., Winberg, J. 'Soothing effect of amniotic fluid smell in newborn infants'. *Early Hum Dev.* 1998 Apr 17;51(1):47-55.
9. Varendi, H., Porter, R.H., Winberg, J. 'Attractiveness of amniotic fluid odor: evidence of prenatal olfactory learning?' *Acta Paediatr.* 1996 Oct;85(10):1223-7.
10. Schaal, B., Marlier, L., Soussignan, R. 'Olfactory function in the human fetus: evidence from selective neonatal responsiveness to the odor of amniotic fluid'. *Behav Neurosci.* 1998 Dec;112(6):1438-49.
11. Marlier, L., Schaal, B., Soussignan, R. 'Neonatal responsiveness to the odor of amniotic and lacteal fluids: a test of perinatal chemosensory continuity'. *Child Dev.* 1998 Jun;69(3):611-23.
12. Marlier, L., Schaal, B., Soussignan, R. 'Bottle-fed neonates prefer an odor experienced in utero to an odor experienced postnatally in the feeding context'. *Dev Psychobiol.* 1998 Sep;33(2):133-45.
13. Orefice, G., Modafferi, N., et al. 'Archaic reflexes in normal elderly people'. *Acta Neurol* 1991 Feb;13(1):19-24.
14. Elkadry, E., Kenton, K., et al. 'Do mothers remember key events during labor?' *Am J Obstet Gynecol* 2003;189:195-200.
15. Wang, F., Li, J., et al. 'The GABA(A) receptor mediates the hypnotic activity of melatonin in rats'. *Pharmacol Biochem Behav* 2003 Feb;74(3):573-8.
16. Tysio, R., Nsardou, R., et al. 'Oxytocin-mediated GABA inhibition during delivery attenuates autism pathogenesis in rodent offspring'. *Science.* 2014 Feb 7;343(6171):675-9. doi: 10.1126/science.1247190.
17. Cohen, M., Roselle, D., Chabner, B., Schmidt, T.J., Lippman, M. 'Evidence for a cytoplasmic melatonin receptor'. *Nature.*

1978; 274:894-895.

18. Sharkey, James Thomas, 'Melatonin Regulation of the Oxytocin System in the Pregnant Human Uterus' (2009). *Electronic Theses, Treatises and Dissertations.* Paper 1791. http://diginole.lib.fsu.edu/etd/1791.

19. Olcese, J., Beesley, S. 'Clinical significance of melatonin receptors in the human myometrium'. *Fertil Steril* 2014 Jul 8. pii: S0015-0282(14)00566-4. doi:10.1016/j.fertnstert.2014.06.020. [Epub ahead of print].

20. Schlabritz-Loutsevitch, N., Hellner, N., Middendorf, R., Muller, D., Olcese, J. 'The human myometrium as a target for melatonin'. *J Clin Endocrinol Metab.* 2003;88(2):908-913.

21. Sharkey, J.T., Puttaramu, R., Word, R.A., Olcese, J. 'Melatonin synergizes with oxytocin to enhance contractility of human myometrial smooth muscle cells'. *J Clin Endocrinol Metab* 2009 Feb;94(2):421-7. doi: 10.1210/jc.2008-1723. Epub 2008 Nov 11.

22. Bagci, S., Berner, A.L., et al. 'Melatonin concentration in umbilical cord blood depends on mode of delivery'. *Early Human Development* 2012; 88(6):369-373

23. Ferguson, J.K.W. 'A study of the motility of the intact uterus at term'. *Surg Gynecol Obstet* 1941. 73: 359-66.

24. Flint, A.P., Forsling, M.L., Mitchell, M.D., Turnbull, A.C. 'Temporal relationship between changes in oxytocin and prostaglandin F levels in response to vaginal distension in the pregnant and puerperal ewe'. *J Reprod Fertil.* 1975 Jun;43(3):551-4.

25. Flint, A.P., Forsling, M.L., Mitchell, M.D. 'Blockade of the Ferguson reflex by lumbar epidural anaesthesia in the parturient sheep: effects on oxytocin secretion and uterine venous prostaglandin F levels'. *Horm Metab Res.* 1978 Nov;10(6):545-7.

26. Newton, N., Foshee, D., Newton, M. 'Experimental inhibition of labor through environmental disturbance'. *Obstetrics and Gynecology* 1967; 371-377.

27. Odent, M. 'The fetus ejection reflex'. *Birth* 1987; 14: 104-105.
28. Newton, N. 'The fetus ejection reflex revisited'. *Birth* 1987; 14: 106-108.
29. Odent, M. 'Fear of death during labour'. *Journal of Reproductive and Infant Psychology* 1991; 9: 43-47.
30. Odent, M. 'The second stage as a disruption of the fetus ejection reflex'. *Midwifery Today* 2000;55:12.
31. Wulf Schiefenhovel. *Childbirth among the Eipos, New Guinea.* Film presented at the Congress of Ethnomedicine. 1978. Gottingen. Germany.
32. https://www.thetimes.co.uk/article/knitting-is-such-a-relief-from-lifes-great-terrors-ng5zcdwxg9h
33. Odent, M. 'Knitting midwives for drugless childbirth?' *Midwifery Today* 2004; vol 71: 21-22.
34. Odent, M. 'Knitting needles, cameras and electronic fetal monitors'. *Midwifery Today* Spring 1996; 37: 14-15.

Chapter Four: In the age of the sorcerer's apprentices

1. Odent, M. 2019. 'Human birth preparation'. In: *The Future of Homo.* Hackensack, NJ: World Scientific.
2. Hoekzema, E., ct al. 2016. 'Pregnancy leads to long-lasting changes in human brain structure'. *Nat Neurosci.* doi: 10.1038/nn.4458.
3. Kivela, A. 1991. 'Serum melatonin during human pregnancy'. *Acta Endocrinol* (Copenh) 124(3): 233–37.
4. Nakamura, Y, et al. 2001. 'Changes of serum melatonin level and its relationship to feto-placental unit during pregnancy'. *J Pineal Res* 30(1): 29–33.
5. Children's National Health System. 2018. 'Placental ALLO levels rise during pregnancy and peak as fetuses approach full term.' www.sciencedaily.com/releases/2018/05/180505091803.htm
6. Ekbom, A., et al. 2000. 'Duration of gestation and prostate cancer risk in offspring.' *Cancer Epidemiol Biomarkers Prev* 9(2): 221–23.

7. Wang, D.H., Ran-Ressler, R., St Leger, J., Nilson, E., Palmer, L., Collins, R., Brenna, J.T. (May 2018). 'Sea Lions Develop Human-like Vernix Caseosa Delivering Branched Fats and Squalene to the GI Tract'. *Scientific Reports*. 8(1): 7478. Bibcode:2018NatSR...8.7478W. doi:10.1038/s41598-018-25871-1. PMC 5945841. PMID 29748625.

8. Odent, M. *Primal Health*. Century Hutchinson. London 1986. Last edition. Clairview Books 2007.

Chapter Five: The shamanic midwife

1. Odent, M. 'Between circular and cul-de-sac epidemiology'. *Lancet* April 15, 2000; vol 9212: p 1371.

2. Malek, A., Blann, E., Mattison, D.R. 'Human placental transport of oxytocin'. *J Matern Fetal Med*. 1996 Sep-Oct;5(5):245-55.

3. Yaakov Beilin, Carol A. Bodian, Jane Weiser, et al. 'Effect of labor epidural analgesia with and without fentanyl on infant breast-feeding: a prospective, randomized, double-blind study'. *Anesthesiology* 2005 Dec;103(6):1211-7. doi: 10.1097/00000542-200512000-00016.

4. Odent, S., Odent, M. 'Primal health research in the age of epigenetic clocks'. *Med Hypotheses* 2019 Dec;133:109403. doi: 10.1016/j.mehy.2019.109403. Epub 2019 Sep 19.

5. Laborit, H. 'Sodium4-hydroxybutyrate'. *Int J Neuropharmacol* 1964;32: 433-451. doi: 10.1016/0028-3908(64)90074-7.

6. Snead, O.C., Gibson, M. 'Gamma-hydroxybutyric acid'. *NEJM* 2005; 352:2721-2732.

7. Santhakumar, V., Wallner, M., Otis, T.S. 'Ethanol acts directly on extrasynaptic subtypes of GABA receptors to increase tonic inhibition'. *Alcohol* 2007; 41 (3): 211–21.

8. Sosa, R., et al. 1980. 'The Effect of a Supportive Companion on Perinatal Problems, Length of Labor, and Mother-Infant Interaction.' *N Engl J Med* 303(11): 597–600.

9. Odent, M. 'Childbirth in the land of Utopia'. Epilogue of: *Childbirth in the age of plastics*. Pinter and Martin, London, 2011.

Chapter Six: Birth at home and birth elsewhere

1. Borghesi, J., Mario, L.C., Rodrigues, M.N., Favaron, P.O., Miglino, M.A. 'Immunoglobulin Transport during Gestation in Domestic Animals and Humans—A Review'. *Open Journal of Animal Sciences*, 2014;4: 323-336.

2. Virella, G., Silveira Nunes, M.A., Tamagnini, G. 'Placental transfer of human IgG subclasses'. *Clin Exp Immunol.* 1972 Mar;10(3):475-8.

3. Pitcher-Wilmott, R.W., Hindocha, P., Wood, C.B. 'The placental transfer of IgG subclasses in human pregnancy'. *Clin Exp Immunol.* 1980 Aug;41(2):303-8.

4. Garty, B.Z., Ludomirsky, A., Danon, Y., J.B. Peter and S.D. Douglas. 'Placental transfer of immunoglobulin G subclasses'. *Clin Diagn Lab Immunol.* 1994 Nov;1(6):667-9.

5. Hashira, S., Okitsu-Negishi, S., Yoshino, K. 'Placental transfer of IgG subclasses in a Japanese population'. *Pediatr Int.* 2000 Aug;42(4):337-42.

6. Coc, C.I., Levine, S., Rosenberg, L.T. 'Effects of age, sex and psychological disturbance on immunoglobin levels in squirrel monkey'. *Developmental Psychobiology* 1988; 21(2): 161-175.

7. Odent, M. 'Home versus hospital birth: the bacteriological perspective'. *Midwifery Today* 2016; 120: 16-18.

8. van Nimwegen, F.A., Penders, J., Stobberingh, E.E., et al. 'Mode and place of delivery, gastrointestinal microbiota, and their influence on asthma and atopy'. *J Allergy Clin Immunol* 2011 Nov;128(5):948-55.e1-3.

9. Odent, M. *The scientification of love*. Free Association Books. London 1999.

10. Kort, R., Caspers, M., de Graaf, A. 'Shaping the oral microbiota through intimate kissing'. *Microbiome.* 2014.

11. Kuitunen, M., Kukkonen, K., Juntunen-Backman, K., et al. 'Probiotics prevent IgE-associated allergy until age 5 years in cesarean-delivered children but not in the total cohort'. *J Allergy Clin Immunol.* 2009 Feb;123(2):335-41. doi: 10.1016/j. jaci.2008.11.019. Epub 2009 Jan 8.

12. Dominguez-Bello, M.G., De Jesus-Laboy, K.M., Shen, N. et al. 'Partial restoration of the microbiota of cesarean-born infants via vaginal microbial transfer'. *Nat Med.* 2016 Mar;22(3):250-3. doi: 10.1038/nm.4039. Epub 2016 Feb 1.
13. Odent, M. 'The fetus ejection reflex'. *Birth* 1987: 14:104-105
14. Odent, M. 'The future of neonatal BCG'. *Medical hypotheses* 2016; 91: 34-36
15. Odent, M. 'Future of BCG'. *Lancet* 1999; 354: 2170

Chapter Seven: Transformations of Homo

1. https://dutchreview.com/author/ceren-spuyman/
2. Laughon, S.K., Branch, D.W., Beaver, J., Zhang, J. 'Changes in labor patterns over 50 years'. *Am J Obstet Gynecol.* 2012 May;206(5):419.e1-9. Epub 2012 Mar 10.
3. Konrath, S.H., O'Brien, E.H., Hsing, C. 'Changes in dispositional empathy in American college students over time: a meta-analysis'. *Pers Soc Psychol Rev.* 2011 May;15(2):180-98. Epub 2010 Aug 5.

Chapter Eight: Can humanity survive socialised access to transcendence?

1. Eaton, S.B., Shostak, M., Konner, M. *The paleolithic prescription.* Harper and Row, New York, 1998.
2. Wulf Schiefenhovel 'Childbirth among the Eipos, New Guinea'. Film presented at the Congress of Ethnomedicine, 1978, Gottingen, Germany.
3. Daniel Everett *Don't sleep, there are snakes.* Profile Books, 2008.
4. Andrew Collins, Gregory L. Little. *Origins of the Gods: Qesem Cave, Skinwalkers, and Contact with Transdimensional Intelligences.* Bear & Company, 2022.
5. Borg, J., Bengt, A., et al. 'The serotonin system and spiritual experiences'. *Am J Psychiatry* 2003. 160(11):1965-9. doi: 10.1176/appi.ajp.160.11.1965
6. Devinsky, J.; Schachter, S. 'Norman Geschwind's contribution to the understanding of behavioral changes in temporal lobe

epilepsy: The February 1974 lecture'. *Epilepsy & Behavior. 15 (4): 417–24.* doi:10.1016/j.yebeh.2009.06.006. PMID 19640791. S2CID 22179745.

7. Zhihao Guo, Baotian Zhao, et al. 'Effective connectivity among the hippocampus, amygdala, and temporal neocortex in epilepsy patients: A cortico-cortical evoked potential study'. *Epilepsy Behav.* 2021 Jan 8;115:107661. doi: 10.1016/j.yebeh.2020.107661.

8. Araujo, L., Ribeiro, O., et al. 'The Role of Existential Beliefs Within the Relation of Centenarians' Health and Well-Being'. *J Relig Health.* 2017 Aug;56(4):1111-1122. DOI: 10.1007/s10943-016-0297-5.

9. Lars Torstam. *Gerotranscendence.* Springer Publishing, 2005.

10. Xavier Patier. *Blaise Pascal. La nuit de l'extase.* Les éditions du Cerf, Paris, 2014.

Chapter Nine: In the beginning was the word

1. Lorber, J. *Die Jugend Jesu.* Stuttgart, Lorber Verlag. Bietigheim/Wurtemberg, 1852.

2. Odent, M. 'Between circular and cul-de-sac epidemiology'. *Lancet* 2000; 355 (April 15): 1371.

3. Jacobson, B., Nyberg, K., Gronbladh, L., et al. 'Opiate addiction in adult offspring through possible imprinting after obstetric treatment'. *BMJ* 1990; 301:1067-70.

4. Frédérick Leboyer. *Pour une naissance sans violence.* Le Seuil. Paris 1974. Available English edition: *Birth without violence.* Pinter & Martin, London 2011.

5. Frédérick Leboyer. *Le Sacre de la naissance.* Phébus, Paris, 1982.

6. Odent, M. 'The early expression of the rooting reflex'. Proceedings of the 5th International Congress of Psychosomatic Obstetrics and Gynaecology, Rome, 1977. London: Academic Press, 1977: 1117-19.

Index

by Michel Odent from Pinter & Martin

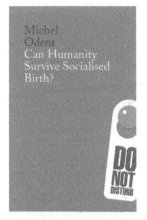

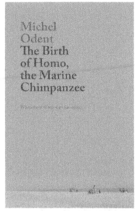

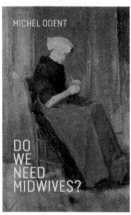

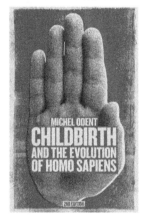

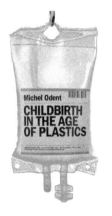

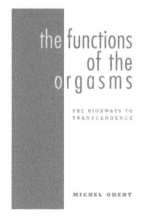

pinterandmartin.com